I0710999

Vegan Cookbook for Athletes

A Plant-Based Diet For High Performance And Muscle Growth At Every Fitness Level; Includes High Protein Recipes For A Healthy And Strong Body Along With Vegan Meal Prep.

© Copyright 2020 - All rights reserved.

The content contained within this book may not be reproduced, duplicated or transmitted without direct written permission from the author or the publisher.
Under no circumstances will any blame or legal responsibility be held against the publisher, or author, for any damages, reparation, or monetary loss due to the information contained within this book. Either directly or indirectly.

Legal Notice:
This book is copyright protected. This book is only for personal use. You cannot amend, distribute, sell, use, quote or paraphrase any part, or the content within this book, without the consent of the author or publisher.

Disclaimer Notice:
Please note the information contained within this document is for educational and entertainment purposes only. All effort has been executed to present accurate, up to date, and reliable, complete information. No warranties of any kind are declared or implied. Readers acknowledge that the author is not engaging in the rendering of legal, financial, medical or professional advice. The content within this book has been derived from various sources. Please consult a licensed professional before attempting any techniques outlined in this book.
By reading this document, the reader agrees that under no circumstances is the author responsible for any losses, direct or indirect, which are incurred as a result of the use of information contained within this document, including, but not limited to, — errors, omissions, or inaccuracies.

Table of Contents

Introduction

Plant foods offer a wide range of advantages over animal foods. They are scientifically recommended for healthy living as they promote a person's wellbeing. By eating plant-based foods, a person is able to reduce the risk of certain illnesses and avoid problems associated with overweight/obesity.

Plant foods are advantageous in their low fat and calorie load. They are also dense in their protein content. Proteins are excellent in helping a person watch weight as they prevent the gaining of body fat. By consuming plant proteins, a person produces more weight limiting hormones. Proteins also help in weight reduction by reducing the feelings of hunger while at the same time increasing the metabolic rate of the body.

By consuming plant products, a person reduces the risk of being overweight. Plants offer excellent sources of fiber, antioxidants, minerals, and vitamins. Plant foods are mainly high in fiber which is helpful in digestion as it limits the amount of sugars absorbed in the digestion process. The fiber in plant foods is also helpful in reducing cholesterol by preventing the absorption of fats in the foods we take. Fiber also helps in preventing constipation in enhancing the digestion of foods. It helps in the stimulation of the various digestive organs to produce important digestive juices. Enough intake of dietary fiber prolongs the amount of time food takes to move through the canal, increasing the absorption of minerals and vitamins in the food. It also prevents diarrhea and excessive hardening of stool.

Research has also confirmed that people who take foods high in fiber are at a lower risk of gaining weight. By consuming foods high in fiber, a person reduces the chances of developing type 2 diabetes. The reason behind the fiber preventing the occurrence of type 2 diabetes is the ability of the fiber to reduce the amounts of sugar the body absorbs maintaining a healthy blood sugar level.

It is also attributed to lowered cholesterol and reduced risk of developing heart disease. The fiber in the digestive system also clumps fats reducing the rate at which they are digested and absorbed in the body. Healthy bacteria in the gut thrive on soluble fiber. The bacteria microbiome feeds on the remains of fermented fiber in the digestive system. These bacteria help in the production of short-chain fatty-acids that help in reducing cholesterol in the body. The short chain fatty-acids also promote good health by reducing inflammation in the body. Inflammation is a risky condition linked to the development of serious illnesses such as cancer among others.

Plant foods reduce the risk of cancers, such as colorectal cancer. While animal foods are found to increase the risk of cancer, plants contain phytochemicals and antioxidants that reduce the risk of developing cancer while at the same time fighting the progress of cancer cells. The fiber found in plant foods is also helpful in detoxification of the body. The detoxification process is aided by both soluble and insoluble fiber. The soluble fiber absorbs the excess hormones and toxins within the body, preventing them from being taken up by the cells. Insoluble fiber works by preventing the absorptions of toxins fond in the foods we consume from the digestive track.

Chapter 1. Athlete Getting Started On A Vegan Diet

Common misunderstandings among many people–even in the health and fitness industry is that anyone who switches to a vegan diet will automatically become super healthy. There are plenty of vegan junk foods out there, such as frozen veggie pizza and non-dairy ice cream, which can really kill your health goals if you eat them all the time. Engaging in healthy foods is the only way you can reap health benefits.

On the other side, certain vegan snacks play a role in keeping you focused. They should be consumed in moderation, sparingly and in small bits.

Decide What a Vegan Diet Means for You

The first step is to make a determination on how to organize your vegan diet to help you move from your present culinary viewpoint. This is really unique, something that ranges from individual to individual. While some people choose not to consume any animal products at all, others make do with tiny bits of dairy or food at times. It really is up to you to decide what and how you want your vegan diet to look like. Perhaps notably, you have to make a large portion of your diet from whole vegan foods.

Understand What You Are Eating

Okay, now that you've made the decision, your next move on your side part requires a lot of study. What do we mean by that? Okay, if this is your first time trying out the vegan diet, the amount of foods containing animal products, particularly packaged foods, will shock you. You will find yourself cultivating the custom of reading tags when shopping. It points out that many pre-packaged foods contain animal products, and you need to keep a close eye on the packaging of the ingredients if you just want to stick to plant products for your new diet. You may have decided to allow a certain number of animal products in your diet; well, you'll just have to look out for foods filled with fats, carbohydrates, salt, preservatives, and other things that may affect your healthy diet.

Find Revamped Versions of Your Favorite Recipes

I'm sure you have plenty of favorite dishes, not necessarily vegan. For most people, leaving everything behind is usually the most difficult part. Nonetheless, there is still a way to meet you halfway. Take some time to think about those things you want that are not based on plants. Think along the lines of taste, shape, consistency, and so on; and search for substitutes throughout the diet based on food plants that can do what you're lacking.

Build a Support Network

Building a new routine is complicated, but it doesn't have to be. Find some friends that are glad to be with you in this lifestyle, or even family members. This will help you stay focused and motivated by having a form of emotional support and openness. You can do fun things like try out and share new recipes with these mates or even hit up restaurants offering a variety of vegan options. You can even go one step further and look up local vegan social media groups to help you expand your knowledge and support network.

Getting to the root of a vegan diet

You can find so many fascinating things to learn and do, but for now I'm going to take you to the basics and ask you which foods to avoid.

Valuable vegetables

You'll find a whole variety of vegetables that you'll really get to know quite well when eating vegan.

If you're new to this, at the beginning, you're likely to stick to tried-and-true, popular veggies because they're going to feel healthy. These vegetables are a good start:

Beets

Carrots

Kale

Parsley, basil, and other herbs

Spinach

Squash

Sweet potatoes

Fantastic fruits

We all love it! You need to get on this train if you haven't because the fruits are delicious; sweet; full of sugar, color, and beautiful vitamins; and so, so good for you.

Apples

Avocado

Bananas

Blueberries

Coconut

Mango

Pineapple

Raspberries

Strawberries

Wonderful whole grains

Consuming whole grains of good quality is a healthy part of a diet based on vegetables. Don't worry; you can still have your pastas and breads, but the key word here is "whole." You don't want the real thing to be polished or stored. When purchasing these items, make sure that the only ingredient is the grain itself. While it is possible to purchase proper whole grains in packaging from the shelf, make sure that you double-check the label to confirm that it is indeed a whole grain (and just a whole grain).

Lovable legumes

It is important to learn to love legumes on a vegan diet as they are a fantastic source of food, protein, and energy. It may take you and your body to get used to them for a while, but they will soon be your friends— especially if you find out how fun it is to consume them in soups, salads, burgers, and other inventive foods. Some of the best things to start with here are:

Black beans

Chickpeas

Kidney beans

Lentils

Split peas

Notable nuts and seeds

A handful of nuts are good. But the thing with eating them on a vegan diet is to make sure they are raw and unsalted. Along with your other delicious vegan foods, you should feel free to eat them in moderation as long as you enjoy them in their natural state. Here's the best to start with:

Almonds

Cashews

Chia seeds

Flaxseeds

Hempseeds

Pumpkin seeds

 Sunflower seeds

Walnuts

Chapter 2. Nutrition Tips for Athletes

Load Up on Carbohydrates: Starches are the critical fuel utilized for the duration of an excessive-strength workout. Proof suggests that adding sugars in your diet improves continuance and execution. On a for-each-calorie premise, starch requirements for athletes are like those for any other person. Explicit proposals for competition rely upon weight and motion kind. On the other hand, that hobby is strenuous and tedious.

Carbs are a competitor's fundamental gasoline. Your frame transforms them into glucose, a type of sugar, and shops it for your muscle groups as glycogen. At the point whilst you work out, your frame modifies glycogen into vitality. On the off chance that you exercise for underneath an hour and a half of, you've got enough glycogen to your muscle tissues, on any occasion, for excessive-pressure physical activities. In case you're exercising longer than that, use any of these techniques:

Sugar stacking for three or four days before an event can assist in growing your glycogen level.

Eat a diet that receives approximately 70% of its energy from sugars, including bread, grains, pasta, natural product, and greens, to perform the finest starch stockpiling.

Upon the advent of a first-rate event, devour your last supper three to four hours earlier than running out, to present your belly time to exhaust.

Abstain from eating sugary or dull foods 30 minutes of beginning a movement; they are able to boost up drying out.

Renew carbs, minerals, and water at some stage in lengthy exercising classes. Eat a tidbit and drink liquid every 15 to twenty minutes.

Refined starches (with sugar or flour) skip swiftly into the moving device, wherein they fuel running muscle tissues.

Get Enough Protein, But Not Too Much: Protein is utilized negligibly for fuel. Its essential capacity is fabricating and keeping up body tissue. Plant-based protein sources are best on the grounds that, in contrast to creature sources, they contain fiber and complex starches.

Protein doesn't give a great deal of fuel to vitality. Be that as it may, you need it to keep up your muscles. Comprehend what you need. The normal individual needs 1.2 to 1.4 grams of protein per kilogram of body weight per day.

Support foods. Getting an excessive amount of protein can put a strain on your kidneys. Rather than protein energies, eat top-notch protein, for example, lean meats, fish, poultry, nuts, beans, eggs, or milk.

Drink up. Milk is perhaps the best food for recuperation after an occasion since it gives a decent parity of protein and starches. Milk additionally has both casein and whey protein. The blend might be especially beneficial for competition. Research shows that whey protein is retained swiftly, which could assist velocity healing following an event. Casein is processed all of the greater steadily, making sure of lengthy haul healing of muscle after an exhausting event. Milk, moreover, has calcium, which is sizeable for retaining up stable bones.

Go Easy on Fat: For long exercises, for instance, long-separation races, your body is going to fats for vitality while sugar assets miss the mark.

Most athletes get the entirety of the fat they need by means of observing the significant wholesome standard to expend for the most segment unsaturated fat from foods, for instance, nuts, avocados, olives, vegetable oils, and oily fish like salmon and fish.

Avoid oily foods upon the appearance of an occasion, taking into account that they can foment your stomach.

Drink Fluids Early and Often: Exceptional exercise, particularly in sweltering climate, can rapidly leave you dried out. Lack of hydration, thusly, can hurt your exhibition and, in extraordinary cases, undermine your life.

One approach to screen hydration is to watch out for the shade of your pee.

Since extraordinary exercise causes you to lose liquid rapidly, it's a smart thought to drink liquids before, just as during, an occasion. Continuance athletes, for example, long-distance runners or long-separation cyclists should drink 8 to 12 ounces of liquid every 10 or 15 minutes during an occasion.

Replace Lost Electrolytes: In case you are likewise dropping an amazing deal of liquid as you sweat, weaken sports activities liquids with equivalent measures of water to get the quality parity of liquid and electrolytes.

Chapter 3. Breakfast Recipes

Chocolate PB Smoothie

Preparation Time: 5 minutes
Cooking Time: 0 minutes
Servings: 4
Ingredients
1 banana
¼ cup rolled oats, or 1 scoop plant protein powder
1 tablespoon flaxseed, or chia seeds
1 tablespoon unsweetened cocoa powder
1 tablespoon peanut butter, or almond or sunflower seed butter
1 tablespoon maple syrup (optional)
1 cup alfalfa sprouts, or spinach, chopped (optional)
½ cup non-dairy milk (optional)
1 cup water
Optional
1 teaspoon maca powder
1 teaspoon cocoa nibs

Directions
Purée everything in a blender until smooth, adding more water (or non-dairy milk) if needed. Add bonus boosters, as desired. Purée until blended.
Nutrition: calories: 474; protein: 13g; total fat: 16g; carbohydrates: 79g; fiber: 18g

Orange french toast

Preparation Time: 15 minutes
Cooking Time: 10 minutes
Servings: 4
Ingredients
3 very ripe bananas
1 cup unsweetened nondairy milk
Zest and juice of 1 orange
1 teaspoon ground cinnamon
¼ Teaspoon grated nutmeg
4 slices french bread
1 tablespoon coconut oil
Directions
In a blender, combine the bananas, almond milk, orange juice and zest, cinnamon, and nutmeg and blend until smooth. Pour the mixture into a 9-by-13-inch baking dish. Soak the bread in the mixture for 5 minutes on each side.
While the bread soaks, heat a griddle or sauté pan over medium-high heat. Melt the coconut oil in the pan and swirl to coat. Cook the bread slices until golden brown on both sides, about 5 minutes each. Serve immediately.

Oatmeal Raisin Breakfast Cookie

Preparation Time: 5 minutes
Cooking Time: 15 minutes
Servings: 2 cookies
Ingredients
½ Cup rolled oats
1 tablespoon whole-grain flour
½ Teaspoon baking powder
1 to 2 tablespoons brown sugar
½ Teaspoon pumpkin pie spice or ground cinnamon (optional)
¼ Cup unsweetened applesauce, plus more as needed
2 tablespoons raisins, dried cranberries, or vegan chocolate chips
Directions
In a medium bowl, stir together the oats, flour, baking powder, sugar, and pumpkin pie spice (if using). Stir in the applesauce until thoroughly combined. Add another 1 to 2 tablespoons of applesauce if the mixture looks too dry (this will depend on the type of oats used).
Shape the mixture into 2 cookies. Put them on a microwave-safe plate and heat on high power for 90 seconds. Alternatively, bake on a small tray in a 350°f oven or toaster oven for 15 minutes. Let cool slightly before eating.
Nutrition (2 cookies): calories: 175; protein: 74g; total fat: 2g; saturated fat:0g; carbohydrates: 39g; fiber: 4g

Berry Beetsicle Smoothie

Preparation Time: 3 minutes
Cooking Time: 0minutes
Servings: 1
Ingredients
½ Cup peeled and diced beets
½ Cup frozen raspberries
1 frozen banana
1 tablespoon maple syrup
1 cup unsweetened soy or almond milk
Directions
Combine all the Ingredients in a blender and blend until smooth.

Blueberry Oat Muffins

Preparation Time: 10 minutes
Cooking Time: 20 minutes
Servings: 12 mufins
Ingredients
2 tablespoons coconut oil or vegan margarine, melted, plus more for preparing the muffin tin
1 cup quick-cooking oats or instant oats
1 cup boiling water
½ Cup nondairy milk
¼ Cup ground flaxseed
1 teaspoon vanilla extract
1 teaspoon apple cider vinegar
1½ cups whole-grain flour
½ Cup brown sugar
2 teaspoons baking soda
Pinch salt
1 cup blueberries

Directions
Preheat the oven to 400°f.
Coat a muffin tin with coconut oil, line with paper muffin cups, or use a nonstick tin.
In a large bowl, combine the oats and boiling water. Stir so the oats soften. Add the coconut oil, milk, flaxseed, vanilla, and vinegar and stir to combine. Add the flour, sugar, baking soda, and salt. Stir until just combined. Gently fold in the blueberries. Scoop the muffin mixture into the prepared tin, about ⅓ cup for each muffin.
Bake for 20 to 25 minutes, until slightly browned on top and springy to the touch. Let cool for about 10 minutes. Run a dinner knife around the inside of each cup to loosen, then tilt the muffins on their sides in the muffin wells so air gets underneath. These keep in an airtight container in the refrigerator for up to 1 week or in the freezer indefinitely.
Nutrition (1muffin): calories: 174; protein: 5g; total fat: 3g; saturated fat:2g; carbohydrates: 33g; fiber: 4g

Quinoa Applesauce Muffins

Preparation Time: 10 minutes
Cooking Time: 15 minutes
Servings: 5
Ingredients
2 tablespoons coconut oil or margarine, melted, plus more for coating the muffin tin
¼ Cup ground flaxseed
½ Cup water
2 cups unsweetened applesauce
½ Cup brown sugar
1 teaspoon apple cider vinegar
2½ cups whole-grain flour
1½ cups cooked quinoa
2 teaspoons baking soda
Pinch salt
½ Cup dried cranberries or raisins
Directions
Preheat the oven to 400°f.
Coat a muffin tin with coconut oil, line with paper muffin cups, or use a nonstick tin. In a large bowl, stir together the flaxseed and water. Add the applesauce, sugar, coconut oil, and vinegar. Stir to combine. Add the flour, quinoa, baking soda, and salt, stirring until just combined. Gently fold in the cranberries without stirring too much. Scoop the muffin mixture into the prepared tin, about ⅓ cup for each muffin.
Bake for 15 to 20 minutes, until slightly browned on top and springy to the touch. Let cool for about 10 minutes. Run a dinner knife around the inside of each cup to loosen, then tilt the muffins on their sides in the muffin wells so air gets underneath. These keep in an airtight container in the refrigerator for up to 1 week or in the freezer indefinitely.
Per serving(1muffin): calories: 387; protein: 7g; total fat: 5g; saturated fat: 2g; carbohydrates: 57g; fiber: 8g

Pumpkin pancakes

Preparation Time: 15 minutes
Cooking Time: 15 minutes
Servings: 4
Ingredients
2 cups unsweetened almond milk
1 teaspoon apple cider vinegar
2½ cups whole-wheat flour
2 tablespoons baking powder
½ Teaspoon baking soda
1 teaspoon sea salt
1 teaspoon pumpkin pie spice or ½ teaspoon ground -cinnamon plus ¼ teaspoon grated
-nutmeg plus ¼ teaspoon ground allspice
½ Cup canned pumpkin purée
1 cup water
1 tablespoon coconut oil

Directions
In a small bowl, combine the almond milk and apple cider vinegar. Set aside.
In a bowl, whisk together the flour, baking powder, baking soda, salt, and pumpkin pie spice. In bowl, combine the almond milk mixture, pumpkin purée, and water, whisking to mix well. Mix the wet Ingredients to the dry Ingredients and fold together until the dry -Ingredients are just moistened.
In a nonstick pan or griddle over medium-high heat, melt the coconut oil and swirl to coat. Pour the batter into the pan ¼ cup at a time and cook until the pancakes are browned, about 5 minutes per side. Serve immediately.

Green breakfast smoothie

Preparation Time: 10 minutes
Cooking Time: 0 minutes
Servings: 2
Ingredients
½ Banana, sliced
2 cups spinach or other greens, such as kale
1 cup sliced berries of your choosing, fresh or frozen
1 orange, peeled and cut into segments
1 cup unsweetened nondairy milk
1 cup ice
Directions
In a blender, combine all the Ingredients.
Starting with the blender on low speed, begin blending the smoothie, gradually increasing blender speed until smooth. Serve immediately.

Blueberry Lemonade Smoothie

Preparation Time: 5 minutes
Cooking Time: 0 minutes
Servings: 1
Ingredients
1 cup roughly chopped kale
¾ Cup frozen blueberries
1 cup unsweetened soy or almond milk
Juice of 1 lemon
1 tablespoon maple syrup
Directions
Combine all the Ingredients in a blender and blend until smooth. Enjoy immediately.

Berry Protein Smoothie

Preparation Time: 5 minutes
Cooking Time: 0 minutes
Servings: 1
Ingredients
1 banana
1 cup fresh or frozen berries
¾ Cup water or nondairy milk, plus more as needed
1 scoop plant-based protein powder, 3 ounces silken tofu, ¼ cup rolled oats, or ½ cup cooked quinoa
Additions
 1 tablespoon ground flaxseed or chia seeds
 1 handful fresh spinach or lettuce, or 1 chunk cucumber
Coconut water to replace some of the liquid
Directions:
In a blender, combine the banana, berries, water, and your choice of protein.
Add any addition Ingredients as desired. Purée until smooth and creamy, about 50 seconds.
Add a bit more water if you like a thinner smoothie.
Nutrition: calories: 332; protein: 7g; total fat: 5g; saturated fat: 1g; carbohydrates: 72g; fiber: 11g

Blueberry and chia smoothie

Preparation Time: 10 minutes
Cooking Time: 0 minutes
Servings: 2
Ingredients
2 tablespoons chia seeds
2 cups unsweetened nondairy milk
2 cups blueberries, fresh or frozen
2 tablespoons pure maple syrup or agave
2 tablespoons cocoa powder
Directions:
Soak the chia seeds in the almond milk for 5 minutes.
In a blender, combine the soaked chia seeds, almond milk, blueberries, maple syrup, and cocoa powder and blend until smooth. Serve immediately.

Green Kickstart Smoothie

Preparation Time: 5 minutes

Cooking Time: 0 minutes

Servings: 1

Ingredients

½ Avocado or 1 banana

½ Cup chopped cucumber, peeled if desired

1 handful fresh spinach or chopped lettuce

1 pear or apple, peeled and cored, or 1 cup unsweetened applesauce

2 tablespoons freshly squeezed lime juice

1 cup water or nondairy milk, plus more as needed

Additions

 ½-Inch piece peeled fresh ginger

1 tablespoon ground flaxseed or chia seeds

½ Cup soy yogurt or 3 ounces silken tofu

 Coconut water to replace some of the liquid

 2 tablespoons chopped fresh mint or ½ cup chopped mango

Directions:

In a blender, combine the avocado, cucumber, spinach, pear, lime juice, and water.

Add any Additions Ingredients as desired. Purée until smooth and creamy, about 50 seconds. Add a bit more water if you like a thinner smoothie.

Nutrition: calories: 263; protein: 4g; total fat: 14g; saturated fat: 2g; carbohydrates: 36g; fiber: 10g

Warm Maple and Cinnamon Quinoa

Preparation Time: 5 minutes
Cooking Time: 15 minutes
Servings: 4
Ingredients
1 cup unsweetened nondairy milk
1 cup water
1 cup quinoa, rinsed
1 teaspoon cinnamon
¼ Cup chopped pecans or other nuts or seeds, such as chia, sunflower seeds, or almonds
2 tablespoons pure maple syrup or agave
Directions:
In a medium saucepan over medium-high heat, bring the almond milk, water, and quinoa to a boil. Lower the heat to medium-low and cover. Simmer until the liquid is mostly absorbed and the quinoa softens, about 15 minutes.
Turn off the heat and allow to sit, covered, for 5 minutes. Stir in the cinnamon, pecans, and syrup. Serve hot.

Warm Quinoa Breakfast Bowl

Preparation Time: 5 minutes
Cooking Time: 0 minutes
Servings: 4
Ingredients
3 cups freshly cooked quinoa
1⅓ cups unsweetened soy or almond milk
2 bananas, sliced
1 cup raspberries
1 cup blueberries
½ Cup chopped raw walnuts
¼ Cup maple syrup
Directions:
Divide the Ingredients among 4 bowls, starting with a base of ¾ cup quinoa, ⅓ cup milk, ½ banana, ¼ cup raspberries, ¼ cup blueberries, and 2 tablespoons walnuts.
Drizzle 1 tablespoon of maple syrup over the top of each bowl.

Banana Bread Rice Pudding

Preparation Time: 5 minutes
Cooking Time: 50 minutes
Servings: 4
Ingredients
1cup brown rice
1½ cups water
1½ cups nondairy milk
3 tablespoons sugar (omit if using a sweetened nondairy milk)
2 teaspoons pumpkin pie spice or ground cinnamon
2 bananas
3 tablespoons chopped walnuts or sunflower seeds (optional)
Directions
In a medium pot, combine the rice, water, milk, sugar, and pumpkin pie spice. Bring to a boil over high heat, turn the heat to low, and cover the pot. Simmer, stirring occasionally, until the rice is soft and the liquid is absorbed. White rice takes about 20 minutes; brown rice takes about 50 minutes.
Smash the bananas and stir them into the cooked rice. Serve topped with walnuts (if using). Leftovers will keep refrigerated in an airtight container for up to 5 days.
Nutrition: calories: 479; protein: 9g; total fat: 13g; saturated fat: 1g; carbohydrates: 86g; fiber: 7g

Apple and cinnamon oatmeal

Preparation Time: 10 minutes
Cooking time:10 minutes
Servings: 2
Ingredients
1¼ cups apple cider
1 apple, peeled, cored, and chopped
⅔ Cup rolled oats
1 teaspoon ground cinnamon
1 tablespoon pure maple syrup or agave (optional)
Directions
In a medium saucepan, bring the apple cider to a boil over medium-high heat. Stir in the apple, oats, and cinnamon.
Bring the cereal to a boil and turn down heat to low. Simmer until the oatmeal thickens, 3 to 4 minutes. Spoon into two bowls and sweeten with maple syrup, if using. Serve hot.

Mango Key Lime Pie Smoothie

Preparation Time: 5 minutes
Cooking Time: 0 minutes
Servings: 1
Ingredients
¼ Avocado
1 cup baby spinach
½ Cup frozen mango chunks
1 cup unsweetened soy or almond milk
Juice of 1 lime (preferably a key lime).
1 tablespoon maple syrup
Directions
Combine all the Ingredients in a blender and blend until smooth. Enjoy immediately.

Spiced orange breakfast couscous

Preparation Time: 10 minutes
Cooking Time: 10 minutes
Servings: 4
Ingredients
3 cups orange juice
1½ cups couscous
1 teaspoon ground cinnamon
¼ Teaspoon ground cloves
½ Cup dried fruit, such as raisins or apricots
½ Cup chopped almonds or other nuts or seeds
Directions
In a small saucepan, bring the orange juice to a boil. Add the couscous, cinnamon, and cloves and remove from heat. Cover the pan with a lid and allow to sit until the -couscous softens, about 5 minutes.
Fluff the couscous with a fork and stir in the dried fruit and nuts. Serve -immediately.

Breakfast parfaits

Preparation Time: 15 minutes
Cooking Time: 0 minutes
Servings: 2
Ingredients
One 14-ounce can coconut milk, refrigerated overnight
1 cup granola
½ Cup walnuts
1 cup sliced strawberries or other seasonal berries
Directions
 Pour off the canned coconut-milk liquid and retain the solids.
 In two parfait glasses, layer the coconut-milk solids, granola, walnuts, and -strawberries.
Serve immediately.

Sweet potato and kale hash

Preparation Time: 10 minutes
Cooking Time: 15 minutes
Servings: 2
Ingredients
1 sweet potato
2 tablespoons olive oil
½ Onion, chopped
1 carrot, peeled and chopped
2 garlic cloves, minced
½ Teaspoon dried thyme
1 cup chopped kale
Sea salt
Freshly ground black pepper
Directions
Prick the sweet potato with a fork and microwave on high until soft, about 5 minutes. Remove from the microwave and cut into ¼-inch cubes.

In a large nonstick sauté pan, heat the olive oil over medium-high heat. Add the onion and carrot and cook until softened, about 5 minutes. Add the garlic and thyme and cook until the garlic is fragrant, about 30 seconds.

Add the sweet potatoes and cook until the potatoes begin to brown, about 7 -minutes. Add the kale and cook just until it wilts, 1 to 2 minutes. Season with salt and pepper. Serve immediately.

Delicious Oat Meal

Preparation Time: 10 minutes
Cooking Time: 6 hours
Servings: 4
Ingredients:
3 cups water
3 cups almond milk
1 and ½ cups steel oats
4 dates, pitted and chopped
1 teaspoon cinnamon, ground
2 tablespoons coconut sugar
½ Teaspoon ginger powder
A pinch of nutmeg, ground
A pinch of cloves, ground
1 teaspoon vanilla extract
Directions:
Put water and milk in your slow cooker and stir.
Add oats, dates, cinnamon, sugar, ginger, nutmeg, cloves and vanilla extract, stir, cover and cook on low for 6 hours.
Divide into bowls and serve for breakfast.
Enjoy!
Nutrition: calories 120, fat 1, fiber 2, carbs 3, protein 5

Breakfast Cherry Delight

Preparation Time: 10 minutes
Cooking Time: 8 hours and 10 minutes
Servings: 4
Ingredients:
2 cups almond milk
2 cups water
1 cup steel cut oats
2 tablespoons cocoa powder
1/3 cup cherries, pitted
¼ Cup maple syrup
½ Teaspoon almond extract
For the sauce:
2 tablespoons water
1 and ½ cups cherries, pitted and chopped
¼ Teaspoon almond extract
Directions:
Put the almond milk in your slow cooker.
Add 2 cups water, oats, cocoa powder, 1/3 cup cherries, maples syrup and ½ teaspoon almond extract.
Stir, cover and cook on low for 8 hours.
In a small pan, mix 2 tablespoons water with 1 and ½ cups cherries and ¼ teaspoon almond extract, stir well, bring to a simmer over medium heat and cook for 10 minutes until it thickens.
Divide oatmeal into breakfast bowls, top with the cherries sauce and serve.
Enjoy!
Nutrition: calories 150, fat 1, fiber 2, carbs 6, protein 5

Crazy Maple and Pear Breakfast

Preparation Time: 10 minutes
Cooking Time: 9 hours
Servings: 2
Ingredients:
1 pear, cored and chopped
½ Teaspoon maple extract
2 cups coconut milk
½ Cup steel cut oats
½ Teaspoon vanilla extract
1 tablespoon stevia
¼ Cup walnuts, chopped for serving
Cooking spray
Directions:
Spray your slow cooker with some cooking spray and add coconut milk.
Also, add maple extract, oats, pear, stevia and vanilla extract, stir, cover and cook on low for 9 hours.
Stir your oatmeal again, divide it into breakfast bowls and serve with chopped walnuts on top.
Enjoy!
Nutrition: calories 150, fat 3, fiber 2, carbs 6, protein 6

Hearty French Toast Bowls

Preparation Time: 10 minutes
Cooking Time: 5 hours
Servings: 4
Ingredients:
1 and ½ cups almond milk
1 cup coconut cream
1 tablespoon vanilla extract
½ Tablespoon cinnamon powder
2 tablespoons maple syrup
¼ Cup spenda
2 apples, cored and cubed
½ Cup cranberries, dried
1 pound vegan bread, cubed
Cooking spray
Directions:
Spray your slow cooker with some cooking spray and add the bread.
Also, add cranberries and apples and stir gently.
Add milk, coconut cream, maple syrup, vanilla extract, cinnamon powder and splenda.
Stir, cover and cook on low for 5 hours.
Divide into bowls and serve right away.
Enjoy!
Nutrition: calories 140, fat 2, fiber 3, carbs 6, protein 2

Tofu Burrito

Preparation Time: 10 minutes
Cooking Time: 8 hours
Servings: 4
Ingredients:
15 ounces canned black beans, drained
2 tablespoons onions, chopped
7 ounces tofu, drained and crumbled
2 tablespoons green bell pepper, chopped
½ Teaspoon turmeric
¾ Cup water
¼ Teaspoon smoked paprika
¼ Teaspoon cumin, ground
¼ Teaspoon chili powder
A pinch of salt and black pepper
4 gluten free whole wheat tortillas
Avocado, chopped for serving
Salsa for serving
Directions:
Put black beans in your slow cooker.
Add onions, tofu, bell pepper, turmeric, water, paprika, cumin, chili powder, a pinch of salt and pepper, stir, cover and cook on low for 8 hours.
Divide this on each tortilla, add avocado and salsa, wrap, arrange on plates and serve.
Enjoy!
Nutrition: calories 130, fat 4, fiber 2, carbs 5, protein 4

Tasty Mexican Breakfast

Preparation Time: 10 minutes
Cooking Time: 2 hours
Servings: 4
Ingredients:
1 cup brown rice
1 cup onion, chopped
2 cups veggie stock
1 red bell pepper, chopped
1 green bell pepper, chopped
4 ounces canned green chilies, chopped
15 ounces canned black beans, drained
A pinch of salt
Black pepper to the taste
For the salsa:
3 tablespoons lime juice
1 avocado, pitted, peeled and cubed
½ Cup cilantro, chopped
½ Cup green onions, chopped
½ Cup tomato, chopped
1 poblano pepper, chopped
2 tablespoons olive oil
½ Teaspoon cumin
Directions:
Put the stock in your slow cooker.
Add rice, onions and beans, stir, cover and cook on high for 1 hour and 30 minutes.
Add chilies, red and green bell peppers, a pinch of salt and black pepper, stir, cover again and cook on high for 30 minutes more.
Meanwhile, in a bowl, mix avocado with green onions, tomato, poblano pepper, cilantro, oil, cumin, a pinch of salt, black pepper and lime juice and stir really well.
Divide rice mix into bowls; top each with the salsa you've just made and serve.
Enjoy!
Nutrition: calories 140, fat 2, fiber 2, carbs 5, protein 5

Divine Carrot Oatmeal

Preparation Time: 10 minutes
Cooking Time: 7 hours
Servings: 3
Ingredients:
2 cups coconut milk
½ Cup old fashioned rolled oats
1 cup carrots, chopped
2 tablespoons agave nectar
1 teaspoon cardamom, ground
A pinch of saffron
Some chopped pistachios
Cooking spray
Directions:
Spray your slow cooker with some cooking spray and add coconut milk.
Also, add oats, carrots, agave nectar, cardamom and saffron.
Stir, cover and cook on Low for 7 hours.
Stir oatmeal again, divide into bowls and serve with chopped pistachios on top.
Enjoy!
Nutrition: calories 140, fat 2, fiber 2, carbs 4, protein 5

Wonderful Blueberry Butter

Preparation Time: 10 minutes
Cooking Time: 6 hours
Servings: 12
Ingredients:
5 cups blueberries puree
2 teaspoons cinnamon powder
Zest from 1 lemon
1 cup coconut sugar
½ Teaspoon nutmeg, ground
¼ Teaspoon ginger, ground
Directions:
Put blueberries in your slow cooker, cover and cook on low for 1 hour.
Stir your berries puree, cover and cook on low for 4 hours more.
Add sugar, ginger, nutmeg and lemon zest, stir and cook on high uncovered for 1 hour more.
Divide into jars, cover them and keep in a cold place until you serve it for breakfast.
Enjoy!
Nutrition: calories 143, fat 2, fiber 3, carbs 3, protein 4

Delicious Pumpkin Butter

Preparation Time: 10 minutes
Cooking Time: 4 hours
Servings: 5
Ingredients:
2 teaspoons cinnamon powder
4 cups pumpkin puree
1 and ¼ cup maple syrup
½ Teaspoon nutmeg
1 teaspoon vanilla extract
Directions:
In your slow cooker, mix pumpkin puree with maple syrup and vanilla extract, stir, cover and cook on high for 4 hours.
Add cinnamon and nutmeg, stir, divide into jars and serve for breakfast!
Enjoy!
Nutrition: calories 120, fat 2, fiber 2, carbs 4, protein 2

Chapter 4. Lunch Recipes

Cauliflower Fried Rice

Preparation Time: 25 minutes
Servings: 2
Ingredients:
5 cups cauliflower florets
3 tablespoons peanut oil, divided into 1 tablespoon and 2 tablespoons
3 scallions, sliced
1 tablespoon grated fresh ginger
1 tablespoon minced garlic
½ cup diced red bell pepper
1 cup trimmed and halved snow peas
1 cup shredded carrots
⅓ cup unsalted roasted cashews
3 tablespoons reduced-sodium soy sauce
1 tablespoon toasted sesame oil
Directions:
Pulse the cauliflower florets in a food processor for about 2 minutes or until it resembles rice. Set aside.
Place a large skillet over high heat and heat 1 tablespoon peanut oil. Add the scallions, ginger and garlic, and saute until the scallions have softened. This should be less than 1 minute. Add the bell pepper, snow peas, and carrots. Saute until the carrots are tender or for about 3 minutes. Transfer this mixture to a plate and set aside.
Add the remaining peanut oil to the skillet and heat. Add the cauliflower rice and saute until softened or for 2 minutes. Return the vegetable mixture and remaining ingredients of cashews, soy sauce, and sesame oil to the skillet.
Serve warm.
Nutrition:
Total fat: 40.6g
Cholesterol: 0mg
Sodium: 1019mg
Total carbohydrates: 39.2g
Dietary fiber: 11.2g
Protein: 14g
Calcium: 147mg
Potassium: 1153mg
Iron: 5mg
Vitamin D: 0mcg

Keto Open-faced Hummus Sandwich

Preparation Time: 5 minutes
Servings: 2
Ingredients:
1 large slice almond bread
4 tablespoons chickpea hummus (See recipe Chapter 5: Sauce and Condiment Recipes: Chickpea Hummus)
4 small baby plum tomatoes, sliced in half
1 cup arugula
1 tablespoon toasted sesame seeds
Olive oil and salt for topping
Directions:
Spread the chickpea hummus over the almond bread.
Top the hummus with plum tomato slices and arugula.
Sprinkle with toasted sesame seeds and finish by drizzling with olive oil and salt.
Slice in half and serve immediately.
Nutrition:
Total fat: 17.2g
Cholesterol: 0mg
Sodium: 293mg
Total carbohydrates: 26.6g
Dietary fiber: 5.7g
Protein: 7.5g
Calcium: 100mg
Potassium: 105mg
Iron: 2mg
Vitamin D: 0mcg

Creamy Keto Butternut Squash Soup

Preparation Time: 1 hour 15 minutes
Servings: 6
Ingredients:
1 lb butternut squash
1 ½ cup coconut milk
4 cups vegetable broth
2 tablespoons avocado oil
6 garlic cloves, minced
2 tablespoons fresh thyme
½ teaspoon cinnamon
⅛ teaspoon nutmeg
Salt and pepper to taste
Directions:
Preheat your oven to 400 degrees F.
Prepare a baking sheet by lining it with parchment paper.
Cut a butternut squash in half lengthwise and remove the seeds. Place the two halves open side up on baking sheet. Drizzle with 1 tablespoon of the avocado oil. Sprinkle with salt and pepper. Flip the 2 halves over, face down.
Roasted butternut squash in the oven for 50 minutes or until it is fork tender.
About 30 minutes into the roasting process, heat the remaining avocado oil in a large pot over medium heat. Add minced garlic, thyme, cinnamon, and nutmeg and saute for about 1 minute or until it becomes fragrant.
Add the coconut oil and vegetable broth to the pot and simmer for 20 minutes or until the squash is completely cooked.
Scoop the squash out of the shells and place into the soup. Puree to a smooth consistency with an immersion blender.
Serve warm. Makes for an especially nourishing meal on snowy and rainy days.
Nutrition:
Total fat: 16g
Cholesterol: 0mg
Sodium: 522mg
Total carbohydrates: 14.8g
Dietary fiber: 3.6g
Protein: 5.7g
Calcium: 77mg
Potassium: 5971mg
Iron: 3mg
Vitamin D: 0mcg

Vegan BLT Sandwich

Preparation Time: 1 hour 45 minutes
Servings: 8
Ingredients:
24 thin slices tempeh (serves as the bacon in the BLT sandwiches)
¼ cup liquid aminos
½ cup of water
2 tablespoons apple cider vinegar
1 teaspoon coconut sugar
½ teaspoon ground cumin
½ teaspoon paprika
Olive oil
To arrange sandwich
16 slices almond or coconut bread
2 ripe avocados
Thick slices of 1 tomato
8 leaves iceberg lettuce
Vegan mayonnaise
Directions:
In a small saucepan, combine the liquid aminos, apple cider vinegar, coconut sugar, cumin, paprika, and water. Bring to a boil over medium heat. Allow to boil for no more than 2 minutes then turn off the heat

Arrange the tempeh slices in a single layer in a casserole dish and pour the liquid aminos marinade over the top. Shake the casserole dish slightly to ensure that all the slices are coated with the marinade. Cover and allow to marinate for at least one hour. Overnight works best.

Preheat your oven to 300 degrees F.

Prepare a baking sheet by lining it with parchment paper and brushing the parchment paper with olive oil.

Drain the tempeh slices and arrange them in a single layer on the prepared baking sheet. Brush the top of the slices with olive oil.

Bake for 15 minutes or until the slices a slightly brown on the edges. Flip the slices and bake for 10 more minutes or until the slices become crisp.

Allow the slices to cool slightly before using.

To arrange the sandwiches, lightly toast the bread slices. Spread one side of the sandwich with vegan mayonnaise once this has been done.

Slice the avocado and arrange slices on top of the vegan mayonnaise-slathered bread slices.

Arrange the tempeh slices, tomato slices, and lettuce over. Top with the other slice of bread.

 Serve immediately.

Nutrition:

Total fat: 23.7g

Cholesterol: 0mg

Sodium: 1045mg

Total carbohydrates: 63.7g

Dietary fiber: 18.5g

Protein: 36.4g

Calcium: 21mg

Potassium: 350mg

Iron: 4mg

Vitamin D: 0mcg

Veggie Pita Pizza

Preparation Time: 20 minutes
Servings: 2
Ingredients:
1 pita bread
⅛ teaspoon dried basil
⅛ teaspoon dried oregano
1 cup tomato sauce
Toppings
3 mushrooms, sliced
⅛ cup chopped yellow onions
⅛ cup chopped green peppers
⅛ cup chopped scallions
Directions:
Preheat your oven to 300 degrees F.
Prepare a small baking sheet by lining it with parchment paper.
Cut the pita bread in half, separating it into two circles.
Spread tomato sauce over each circle. Sprinkle with the basil and oregano. Arrange the toppings next.
Bake for 10 minutes. Alternately, this can be heated in a toaster oven for 5 minutes at 250 degrees F.
Serve warm.
Nutrition:
Total fat: 1.2g
Cholesterol: 0mg
Sodium: 817mg
Total carbohydrates: 31.4g
Dietary fiber: 6.7g
Protein: 6.5g
Calcium: 65mg
Potassium: 667mg
Iron: 4mg
Vitamin D: 97mcg

Black Bean Salad

Preparation Time: 10 minutes
Servings: 4
Ingredients:
2 16-oz cans of black beans, drained and rinsed well
2 cup fresh corn
1 large tomato, chopped
½ cup yellow onion, chopped
1 cup pecans, chopped
¼ cup cilantro chopped
Juice and zest of 1 small lime
Balsamic vinegar to taste
Directions:
To a large bowl, add the black beans, corn, tomato, yellow onion, and pecans, and mix well.
Add the cilantro, juice and zest of the lime and balsamic. Mix again.
Can be served alone or as a side to a sandwich or meal.
Nutrition:
Total fat: 14.1g
Cholesterol: 0mg
Sodium: 706mg
Total carbohydrates: 51.7g
Dietary fiber: 17.7g
Protein: 15.9g
Calcium: 89mg
Potassium: 981mg
Iron: 4mg
Vitamin D: 97mcg

Jackfruit Veggie Tacos

Preparation Time: 20 minutes
Servings: 8
Ingredients:
1 10-oz package jackfruit
8 corn tortillas, warmed
1 ripe avocado, chopped
¼ cup plain unsweetened almond milk
2 tablespoons olive oil
3 tablespoons lime juice
½ teaspoon salt
1 medium tomato, diced
¼ cup fresh cilantro, chopped
2 tablespoons onion, diced
1 tablespoon jalapeno pepper, diced
1 cup salt-free pinto beans, rinsed
1 cup romaine lettuce, shredded
Directions:
Add the avocado, almond milk, 2 tablespoons of lime juice, and ¼ teaspoon of salt into a blender. Blend until a creamy consistency is reached. Scrape down the sides of the blender if necessary

In a medium bowl, combine the remaining lime juice, 1 tablespoon of olive oil, the remaining salt, tomato, cilantro, onions, and jalapeno. Combine well.

Heat up the remaining olive oil in a large nonstick skillet over. Add the jackfruit and pinto beans and cook for up to 3 minutes or until heated through. Stir occasionally.

Serve the pinto beans and jackfruit in corn tortillas topped with the avocado mixture and lettuce.

Nutrition:
Total fat: 9.5g
Cholesterol: 0mg
Sodium: 167mg
Total carbohydrates: 29g
Dietary fiber: 6.1g
Protein: 4.6g
Calcium: 49mg
Potassium: 4361mg
Iron: 1mg
Vitamin D: 0mcg

Sauteed Veggies in Spicy Garlic Chili Sauce

Preparation Time: 15 minutes

Servings: 2

Ingredients:

½ cup red bell peppers, chopped

½ cup green bell peppers, chopped

½ cup yellow bell peppers, chopped

1 red onion, chopped

½ cup white mushrooms, sliced

1 cup broccoli florets

½ cup baby corn, chopped

½ cup sugar snap peas

¼ cup leeks, sliced

1 teaspoon sesame seeds

1 teaspoon of olive oil

2 tablespoons spicy garlic chili sauce (See recipe Chapter 5: Sauce and Condiment Recipes: Spicy Garlic Chili Sauce)

1 1/2 cup water

5 basil leaves

Directions:

Heat the olive oil in a large, nonstick skillet over medium heat. Add the sesame seeds and basil leaves and saute for 10 seconds.

Add leeks and red onions and saute for 1 minute.

Add all bell peppers and saute for 1 minute.

Add the rest of the vegetables and saute for 2 minutes.

Add the water and garlic chili sauce. Stir. Cover the pot and cook for 4 minutes.

Can be served as is or over rice.

Nutrition:

Total fat: 3.4g

Cholesterol: 0mg

Sodium: 40mg

Total carbohydrates: 25.7g

Dietary fiber: 5.5g

Protein: 5.3g

Calcium: 63mg

Potassium: 613mg

Iron: 3mg

Vitamin D: 63mcg

Raw Mushroom Walnut Lettuce Wraps

Preparation Time: 3 hours 15 minutes
Servings: 5
Ingredients:
3 cups mushrooms, roughly chopped
3 tablespoons liquid aminos
2 tablespoons maple syrup
1 teaspoon apple cider vinegar
2 cups walnuts
4 cups water
1 cup quinoa, cooked
½ teaspoon cumin
½ teaspoon smoked paprika
½ teaspoon coriander
½ teaspoon chipotle powder
⅓ cup parsley, chopped
1 cup cherry tomatoes, quartered
1 small avocado, sliced
5 large butter lettuce leaves
Salt and pepper to taste
Directions:
Mix liquid aminos, maple syrup, and apple cider vinegar in a small bowl.
Place mushroom pieces in a medium sealable bowl. Pour the maple syrup mixture over the mushrooms. Seal the bowl and shake so that the mushrooms are coated with the mixture.
Place the bowl in the refrigerator and let marinade for 3 hours. Shake occasionally to coat mushrooms.
While the mushroom marinade, cover the walnuts in water and let soak for 3 hours.
Drain and rinse the walnuts. Place in a food processor. Pulse until a chunky texture is achieved.
Add the marinated mushrooms and parsley to the food processor. Pulse until the mushrooms and parsley are well incorporated.
Stir in all spices, quinoa, salt, and pepper.
To assemble wraps, place the mixture in the lettuce leaves. Top with tomatoes pieces and avocado slices.
Sprinkle with salt and pepper. Serve.
Nutrition:
Total fat: 40.4g

Cholesterol: 0mg
Sodium: 133mg
Total carbohydrates: 39.5g
Dietary fiber: 9.7g
Protein: 19.8g
Calcium: 74mg
Potassium: 938mg
Iron: 6mg
Vitamin D: 151mcg

Avocado Arugula Salad

Preparation Time: 10 minutes
Servings: 6
Ingredients:
2 large ripe, firm avocados, diced into large chunks
½ cup baby arugula, roughly chopped
¼ cup red onions, diced
1 cup cherry tomatoes, halved
1 cup grape tomatoes, halved
6 basil leaves, thinly sliced
    2 tablespoons orange olive vinaigrette
Directions:
Place all the avocado pieces, arugula, onions, tomatoes, and basil leaves in a large bowl.
Toss with vinaigrette and serve. Squeeze fresh lemon juice over the avocado chunks if you
plan to serve later. This prevents the avocado from turning brown.
Nutrition:
Total fat: 14.7g
Cholesterol: 0mg
Sodium: 123mg
Total carbohydrates: 8.6g
Dietary fiber: 5.1g
Protein: 1.7g
Calcium: 17mg
Potassium: 418mg
Iron: 1mg
Vitamin D: 0mcg

Keto Avocado Kale Salad

Preparation Time: 15 minutes
Servings: 4
Ingredients:
10 Tuscan kale leaves
2 teaspoons of olive oil
2 teaspoons of sesame oil
1 teaspoon fresh ginger, grated
1 garlic cloves, grated
A pinch of salt
½ cup snow peas, chopped
1 ripe avocado, cliced
⅓ cup scallions, shopped
1 teaspoon lemon zest
2 teaspoons balsamic vinegar
2 teaspoons liquid aminos
Directions:
Wash, rinse, and dry the kale leaves. Remove the stems with a knife. Slice the kale leaves into small pieces.
Add the kale pieces to a large bowl. Add the olive oil, sesame oil, ginger, garlic, and salt. Toss and ensure the kale leaves are thoroughly coated.
Add all the remaining ingredients and toss again. Refrigerate for 5 minutes and serve chilled.
Nutrition:
Total fat: 5.8g
Cholesterol: 0mg
Sodium: 56mg
Total carbohydrates: 4.2g
Dietary fiber: 1.9g
Protein: 1.2g
Calcium: 27mg
Potassium: 197mg
Iron: 1mg
Vitamin D: 0mcg

Spaghetti Squash with Mushrooms and Tomatoes

Preparation Time: 60 minutes
Servings: 6
Ingredients:
1 spaghetti squash
1 cup mushrooms, sliced
2 cups tomatoes, diced
4 garlic cloves, minced
¼ cup onions, chopped
¼ cup pine nuts, toasted
1 tablespoon fresh basil, finely chopped
3 tablespoons olive oil
Salt and pepper to taste
Directions:
Wash and dry the spaghetti squash. Cut into two halves. Pierce the spaghetti squash with a knife several times. Place the spaghetti squash in a shallow baking dish which has about 1 inch of water and bake for up to 45 minutes or until it is soft enough to pierce with the knife easily.
When the squash is cool enough to handle, scoop out the seeds and stringy bits. Shred with a fork and set the spaghetti strands aside.
Heat olive oil in a nonstick skillet over medium heat. Add onions and mushrooms and saute for 4 minutes.
Add garlic and saute for 2 minutes or until fragrant. Do not let garlic brown.
Add tomatoes and cooked spaghetti squash. Cook and stir until the squash is hot and vegetables are evenly distributed.
Remove from heat. Toss with fresh basil and pine nuts. Season with salt and pepper. Serve warm.
Nutrition:
Total fat: 11.5g
Cholesterol: 0mg
Sodium: 19mg
Total carbohydrates: 10.4g
Dietary fiber: 1.2g
Protein: 2.4g
Calcium: 32mg
Potassium: 321mg
Iron: 1mg
Vitamin D: 42mcg

Asian Coleslaw

Preparation Time: 15 minutes
Servings: 10
Ingredients:
6 cups red cabbage, thinly sliced
6 cups green cabbage, thinly sliced
¾ cup shallots, sliced
1 cup cilantro, roughly chopped
2 cups carrots, shredded
1 teaspoon sesame oil
1 tablespoon olive oil
1 tablespoon maple syrup
1 tablespoon apple cider vinegar
2 teaspoons of soy sauce
1 tablespoon rice wine vinegar
2 tablespoons of almond butter
1 garlic clove, minced
½ teaspoon of ginger, grated
¼ teaspoon cayenne pepper
Juice and zest of one small lime
Salt and pepper to taste
Directions:
To make Asian coleslaw dressing, place olive oil, sesame oil, maple syrup, apple cider vinegar, soy sauce, rice wine vinegar, almond butter, garlic, ginger, cayenne pepper, juice and zest of lime, salt, and pepper in a small blender, and blend until a smooth consistency is achieved.

Place the remaining ingredients in a large bowl. Pour the dressing into the bowl. Mix thoroughly.

Refrigerate for at least one hour for the flavors to marinade. Serve chilled.

Nutrition:
Total fat: 3.8g
Cholesterol: 0mg
Sodium: 93mg
Total carbohydrates: 11.7g
Dietary fiber: 3.1g
Protein: 2.4g
Calcium: 50mg
Potassium: 302mg
Iron: 1mg
Vitamin D: 0mcg

Keto Broccoli Fried Rice

Preparation Time: 15 minutes
Servings: 3
Ingredients:
4 cups broccoli florets
1 tablespoon avocado oil
1 tablespoon liquid aminos
1 ½ teaspoon sesame oil
1 tablespoon garlic ,finely chopped
¼ cup cilantro, chopped
2 tablespoons scallions chopped
2 teaspoons of lime juice
½ teaspoon ginger, grated
Sliced almonds for topping
Salt and pepper to taste
Directions:
Add the broccoli florets to a food processor and pulse until a rice-like texture is achieved. Scrape down sides of bowl if necessary.
Add olive oil to a nonstick skillet and place over medium heat. Add riced broccoli and garlic, and saute for 1 minute.
Add liquid aminos, sesame oil, salt, and pepper. Saute for 2 more minutes or until the broccoli achieves a bright green color but is not mushy.
Turn off the heat and add ginger and lime juice. Stir to infuse flavors.
Top with scallions, cilantro and sliced almonds. Serve.
Nutrition:
Total fat: 2.4g
Cholesterol: 0mg
Sodium: 67mg
Total carbohydrates: 17.2g
Dietary fiber: 1.6g
Protein: 2g
Calcium: 22mg
Potassium: 113mg
Iron: 1mg
Vitamin D: 0mcg

Stuffed Tomatoes

Preparation Time: 50 minutes

Servings: 6

Ingredients:

6 large beefsteak tomatoes

¼ cup red onion, diced

1 bell pepper, diced

1 tablespoon olive oil

4 garlic cloves, minced

1 block extra firm tofu, pressed

1 ½ cup cooked black beans, rinsed and drained

1 ½ cup corn, rinsed and drained

2 tablespoons tomato paste

2 tablespoons chili powder

1 teaspoon smoked paprika

1 teaspoon cumin

1 tablespoon lime juice

½ cup fresh cilantro, chopped

Salt and pepper to taste

Directions:

Preheat your oven to 400 degrees F.

Add olive oil to a large nonstick skillet. Place over medium heat. Saute onions and bell peppers until the onions become translucent. Add garlic, chili powder, paprika, cumin, and tomato paste. Saute for 3 minutes.

Add tofu and mix. Cover the pan and cooked for 10 minutes on low heat. Stir occasionally. As the filling cooks, cut the tops of the tomatoes and scoop out the seeds and guts. Sprinkle each tomato with salt and pepper to season.

After the 10 minutes are up, remove the lid and add black beans and corn. Stir and cook until this becomes warm.

Remove the filling from the heat. Add cilantro and lime juice. Stir to combine.

Stuff the tomatoes with good feeling and arrange the tomatoes on a casserole dish.

Bake for 15 minutes or until the tomatoes are blistered. Serve warm. Leftovers can be reserved in the refrigerator or freezer.

Nutrition:
Total fat: 5g
Cholesterol: 0mg
Sodium: 52mg
Total carbohydrates: 50.5g
Dietary fiber: 12.5g
Protein: 15.5g
Calcium: 126mg
Potassium: 1455mg
Iron: 5mg
Vitamin D: 0mcg

Tomato Sandwiches

Preparation Time: 5 minutes
Servings: 2
Ingredients:
2 medium heirloom tomatoes
4 vegan cheese slices
4 slices almond bread (or any gluten-free, dairy-free bread that you prefer)
Pesto sauce(see recipe Chapter 5: Sauces and Condiments: Vegan Garden Pesto Sauce)
4 lettuce leaves
Directions:
Slice the tomatoes.
To assemble sandwiches, layer lettuce, tomato slices, and vegan cheese on one slice of bread. Drizzle with pesto sauce. Top with another bread slice. Repeat with the remaining slices of bread. Can be served cold or pressed like a normal grilled cheese sandwich and served warm.
Nutrition:
Total fat: 2.4g
Cholesterol: 0mg
Sodium: 67mg
Total carbohydrates: 17.2g
Dietary fiber: 1.6g
Protein: 2g
Calcium: 22mg
Potassium: 113mg
Iron: 1mg
Vitamin D: 0mcg

Dulse, Tomato & Lettuce Sandwiches

Preparation Time: 10 minutes
Servings: 2
Ingredients
4 slices whole-grain bread
4 tbsp. mayonnaise, vegan
½ cup Dulse seaweed
1 tomatoes
½ cup lettuce
Directions
Over medium heat in a large skillet, dry fry the Dulse until the leaves turn greenish, (black=burnt) for a few minutes. Let it cool at room temperature
In the meantime, make the tomato slice and toast bread, if desired. Spread mayonnaise over the bread. Top the bread with Dulse, tomato, and lettuce. Season with pepper and salt, if desired.
Nutrition: 224.2 Calories, 7.7 g Total Fat, 7.2 mg Cholesterol, 34.6 g Carbohydrate, 2.2 g Fiber, 5.2 g Protein

Sugar and Spice Almonds

Preparation Time: 15 minutes
Servings: 2 cups
Ingredients
2 cups whole almonds
3 tbsp. light corn syrup
⅓ cup granulated sugar (or vegan sugar)
½ tsp. nutmeg, freshly ground
4 tsp. ground cinnamon
Directions
Preheat your oven at 350 F/175 C.
Spray a baking sheet (preferably large) with cooking spray (non-sticking), or put a few drops of oil & use a paper towel to spread it evenly.
Combine sugar, nutmeg, and cinnamon in a small dish and keep it aside.
Combine the corn syrup with the almonds until the almonds are well coated in a different bowl; sprinkle sugar over the almonds and stir. Ensure it gets mixed in evenly.
Put the coated almonds on the greased baking sheet & bake until the almonds are browned & bubbly, approximately 15 minutes; remove the almonds from the oven.
Let the almonds cool down on the baking sheet at the room temperature, stirring to separate the nuts and to prevent sticking.
You may even store the crispy almonds in an airtight container, not for that long!
Nutrition: 1063.8 Calories, 72.8 g Total Fat, 0 mg Cholesterol, 90.8 g Carbohydrate, 19.5 g Fiber, 30.6 g Protein

Roasted Green Beans

Preparation Time: 25 minutes
Servings: 6
Ingredients
2 pounds' green beans
2 tbsp. olive oil
1 tsp. kosher salt
½ tsp. ground pepper, fresh
Directions
Preheat your oven at 400F/200 C.
Wash and rinse the green beans (make sure that the beans are neat, dry well).
Arrange the green beans on a jelly roll pan & drizzle olive oil over it.
Sprinkle with pepper and salt to taste.
Coat the beans evenly using your hands and then spread the beans out into one layer.
Roast until beans are somewhat shriveled and fairly brown in the spots, approximately half an hour; don't forget to turn the beans after every 10 to 15 minutes.
Serve at room temperature or hot.
Nutrition: 100.9 Calories, 3.9 g Total Fat, 0 mg Cholesterol, 16 g Carbohydrate, 6.2 g Fiber, 4.2 g Protein

Cauliflower Popcorn

Preparation Time: 70 minutes
Servings: 4
Ingredients
1 head cauliflower
4 tbsp. olive oil
1 tsp. salt, to taste
Directions
Preheat your oven at 425 F/220 C.
Trim the head of the cauliflower and discard the thick stems and core; cut the florets and make Ping-Pong balls size pieces.
Mix the salt and olive oil together in a large bowl, whisk and then put the cauliflower pieces & toss thoroughly.
For easy cleanup, line a baking sheet with parchment then spread the cauliflower pieces on the sheet & roast until most of the pieces have turned golden brown, approximately an hour, turning 4 or 5 times.
Nutrition: 156.1 Calories, 13.9 g Total Fat, 0 mg Cholesterol, 7.3 g Carbohydrate, 2.9 g Fiber, 2.8 g Protein

Onions and Spinach

Preparation Time: 25 minutes
Servings: 4
Ingredients
3 tbsp. light olive oil
1 red onion, large & thinly sliced
1-pound spinach leaves, fresh, cleaned & stems removed
1 tbsp. lemon juice, fresh
pepper and salt (as per taste)
Directions
Heat olive oil in a large skillet.
Add onions, only when the oil gets hot, ensure it's not smoking.
Sauté, until the onion is caramelized, stirring constantly, approximately 15 min let some
of the onion get crisp and quite dark.
Now put the spinach leaves, for a minute or two & stir until just wilted.
Now put in the lemon juice, pepper & salt and mix with the prepared dish.
Serve.
Nutrition: 131.4 Calories, 10.6 g Total Fat, 0 mg Cholesterol
7.9 g Carbohydrate, 3.2 g Fiber, 3.7 g Protein

Zucchini Noodle Salad

Preparation Time: 35 minutes
Servings: 4
Ingredients:
2 zucchinis
3 carrots
1 cup spinach, thinly sliced
3 tablespoons soy sauce
¼ cup natural smooth peanut butter
¼ cup peanuts roughly chopped
2 tablespoons lime juice
1 tablespoon maple syrup
¼ cup cilantro finely chopped
   Water
Directions:
Using a spiralizer, spiralize the zucchini and carrots into noodles. Add the spiralized noodles and the sliced cabbage to a large bowl.
Place peanut butter in a small microwave safe bowl and microwave for 20 seconds. Stir to achieve a smooth consistency.
Add lemon juice, maple syrup, and soy sauce to peanut butter. Whisk to combine. Add water if needed to achieve a smooth salad dressing-like consistency.
Add peanut sauce, peanuts, and cilantro to veggie noodles. Toss to combine.
Refrigerate for 30 minutes and serve chilled.
Nutrition:
Total fat: 27.7g
Cholesterol: 0mg
Sodium: 927mg
Total carbohydrates: 20.2g
Dietary fiber: 7.6g
Protein: 19.7g
Calcium: 55mg
Potassium: 567mg
Iron: 1mg
Vitamin D: 0mcg

Quinoa Veggie Chopped Salad

Preparation Time: 25 minutes
Servings: 6
Ingredients:
2 cups quinoa, cooked
1 red bell pepper, chopped
1 carrot, chopped
1 medium cucumber, chopped
1 cup arugula
1 cup cherry tomatoes, halved
½ cup pumpkin seeds
1 cup corn
½ cup white balsamic vinegar
1 tablespoon maple syrup
¼ cup olive oil
1 tablespoon lemon juice
1 garlic clove, grated
Salt and pepper to taste
Directions:
Combine quinoa, bell pepper, carrots, cucumber, tomatoes, corn, arugula, and pumpkin seeds in a large bowl.
To make balsamic vinaigrette, whisk together white balsamic vinegar, garlic, lemon juice, maple syrup, salt, and pepper. Slowly drizzle in olive oil while continuously whisking.
Pour white balsamic vinaigrette over the chopped salad. Toss to combine and refrigerate for 30 minutes. Serve chilled.
Nutrition:
Total fat: 17.6g
Cholesterol: 0mg
Sodium: 22mg
Total carbohydrates: 51.5g
Dietary fiber: 6.3g
Protein: 12.7g
Calcium: 58mg
Potassium: 735mg
Iron: 5mg
Vitamin D: 0mcg

Spinach Mushroom Tofu Wraps

Preparation Time: 50 minutes
Servings: 4
Ingredients:
1 block firm tofu
2 cups mushrooms, sliced
½ cup spinach, frozen
½ cup cherry tomatoes
½ teaspoon curry powder
½ teaspoon turmeric
2 teaspoons canola oil
½ teaspoon salt
2 vegan tortillas
   4 tablespoon chickpea hummus
Directions:
Add canola oil to a medium skillet and place over medium heat. Crumble the tofu and add to skillet. Scramble.
Add turmeric, salt, and curry powder. Mix well so that tofu gets an evenly distributed yellow color. Saute for 3 minutes.
Add sliced mushrooms and spinach and cook for 10 minutes.
To arrange tortillas, warm tortillas in a pan then spread 2 tablespoons of hummus on the tortilla. Top with tofu mixture and tomatoes. Fold wrap and serve.
Nutrition:
Total fat: 11.3g
Cholesterol: 0mg
Sodium: 781mg
Total carbohydrates: 32.8g
Dietary fiber: 2g
Protein: 9.9g
Calcium: 74mg
Potassium: 230mg
Iron: 2mg
Vitamin D: 126mcg

Vegan Spring Rolls

Preparation Time: 10 minutes
Servings: 8
Ingredients:
8 rice paper wrappers
8 lettuce leaves
1 red bell pepper, thinly sliced
1 cup red cabbage, thinly sliced
2 medium carrots, thinly sliced
¼ cup fresh cilantro, chopped
¼ cup fresh basil, chopped
3 oz rice noodles, cooked
Almond dipping sauce for dipping
Directions:
To soften the rice papers, fill a large bowl with warm water and dip each rice paper into it for 5 to 10 seconds. Do not hold the rice paper in there longer because it will break apart. Layer the rice papers on a flat surface.

Beginning at one end of one rice paper, layer veggies by starting with lettuce and adding cabbage, bell peppers, carrots, rice noodles, cilantro, and basil on top. Gently fold the rice paper so that the veggies are tucked inside.

Serve immediately with almond dipping sauce. Can be wrapped in plastic wrap and refrigerated to preserve for a later serving.

Nutrition:
Total fat: 2.4g
Cholesterol: 0mg
Sodium: 67mg
Total carbohydrates: 17.2g
Dietary fiber: 1.6g
Protein: 2g
Calcium: 22mg
Potassium: 113mg
Iron: 1mg
Vitamin D: 0mcg

Chapter 5. Dinner Recipes

Beans and Button Mushrooms "Stew"

Ingredients
4 Tbsp olive oil
1 cup chopped onion
1 tsp minced garlic
1 lb fresh button mushrooms, sliced
3/4 tsp dried thyme, crushed
1 tsp red paprika
2 cups vegetable broth
1 can (11 oz) tomatoes crushed
2 can (15 oz) white beans, drained
Salt and ground black pepper to taste
Directions:
Heat olive oil in a pot over medium-high heat.
Add onion, garlic, mushrooms, thyme, and red paprika; sauté for about 4 to 5 minutes.
Pour the vegetable broth and tomatoes, and bring to a boil.
Reduce heat to medium, cover and cook for 15 to 17 minutes
Add the beans and stir; cook for a further 2 to 3 minutes.
Remove from heat and adjust the salt and pepper to taste.
Serve warm.
Ready in Preparation Time: 35 minutes
Nutrition Facts
Percent daily values based on the Reference Daily Intake (RDI) for a 2000 calorie diet.
Nutrition:
Calories 347.87
Calories From Fat95.33
% Daily Value
Total Fat 10.82g
Saturated Fat 1.65g 8%
Cholesterol 0.62mg <1%
Sodium 524.34mg
Potassium 1221.5mg
Total Carbohydrates 49g
Fiber 10.43g
Sugar 4.77g
Protein 16.5g

Boosting Black Beans and Avocado Salad

Ingredients
2 can (11 oz) black beans drained
1 avocado cored, cut into cubes
3/4 cup green onions finely chopped
1 cup corn kernels, drained
1 tomato sliced
1 clove garlic finely sliced
1 red bell pepper cut in strips
1 pear cut into cubes
1/2 cup olive oil
1/3 cup fresh lime juice
1/4 tsp salt and ground black pepper to taste
1/2 cup chopped cilantro fresh
2 Tbsp parsley finely chopped

Directions:
In a large and deep bowl combine together black beans, avocado, green onion, corn, tomato, garlic, pear, and bell pepper.
In a separate bowl, combine all remaining ingredients and pour over black bean mixture.
Toss to combine well.
Taste and adjust salt and pepper to taste.
Serve immediately.
Servings: 4
Ready in Preparation Time: 15 minutes
Nutrition Facts
Percent daily values based on the Reference Daily Intake (RDI) for a 2000 calorie diet.
Nutrition:
Calories 561.44
Calories From Fat305.11
% Daily Value
Total Fat 34.91g
Saturated Fat 4.87g
Cholesterol 0mg 0%
Sodium 542mg
Potassium 1072.47mg
Total Carbohydrates 54.76g
Fiber 17.1g
Sugar 9.3g
Protein 13.88g

Brown Rice Pasta Salad with Apple Juice Sauce

Ingredients
1 lb Brown rice pasta
1 can (11 oz) corn boiled, drained
1/2 cup chopped red onion
1 cup carrots, shredded
2 roasted red peppers cut into slices or cubes
2 cups mushrooms, sliced
1/2 cup olive oil
1/2 cup apple juice canned or bottled
1/3 cup chopped fresh basil
Salt and freshly ground black pepper
Directions:
Prepare pasta according to package directions.
Drain pasta and rinse with cold water.
Add brown rice pasta into a large salad bowl together with corn, red onion, carrot, peppers, and mushrooms.
In a separate bowl, whisk together olive oil, apple juice, basil, and salt and pepper.
Pour olive oil sauce over the pasta salad; toss to combine well.
Taste and adjust the salt and pepper to taste.
Serve or keep refrigerated.
Servings: 4
Ready in Preparation Time: 15 minutes
Nutrition Facts
Percent daily values based on the Reference Daily Intake (RDI) for a 2000 calorie diet.
Nutrition:
Calories 745.1
Calories From Fat247.48
% Daily Value
Total Fat 28g
Saturated Fat 4g
Cholesterol 0mg 0%
Sodium 185.64mg 8%
Potassium 517.75mg
Total Carbohydrates 105.67g
Fiber 9.16g
Sugar 6.4g
Protein 19g

Garlic -Potato Puree

Ingredients
6 potatoes peeled and halved
Water for cooking
8 cloves of garlic, cleaned
3/4 cup olive oil
2 Tbsp white wine vinegar
Kosher salt and ground white pepper
2 Tbsp fresh parsley chopped for serving

Directions:
Peel, cut into halves and rinse potatoes.

Cook potatoes in boiling water until tender or about 20 to 25 minutes for halved potatoes.

Transfer potatoes in a colander and drain well.

Add garlic and olive oil, some salt and pepper in a high-speed blender; blend until combined.

Add potatoes and continue to blend until well combined.

Remove mixture to a bowl, pour the vinegar and stir with a spoon.

Taste and adjust salt and pepper to taste.

Sprinkle with chopped parsley and serve!

Keep refrigerated.

Servings: 6

Ready in Preparation Time: 35 minutes

Nutrition Facts

Percent daily values based on the Reference Daily Intake (RDI) for a 2000 calorie diet.

Nutrition:

Calories 413.34

Calories From Fat240.45

% Daily Value

Total Fat 27.21g

Saturated Fat 3.79g

Cholesterol 0mg 0%

Sodium 15.23mg <1%

Potassium 919mg

Total Carbohydrates 39.44g

Fiber 4.77g

Sugar 2.5g

Protein 5g

High Protein Soybean Pasta with Basil

Ingredients
1/2 lb soybean pasta
1 can (11 oz) white bean cooked
4 tsp olive oil
4 tsp garlic finely chopped
1 can (15 oz) tomato crushed
1 can (11 oz) tomato paste
2 tsp dried oregano
Salt and ground black pepper to taste
1/2 cup fresh basil chopped
Directions:
Prepare soybean pasta according to package directions; drain.
Mash white beans in a blender; set aside.
Heat the oil in a saucepan over medium-high heat.
Sauté garlic until soft (do not burn it).
Add crushed tomatoes and beans, tomato paste, oregano, salt, and pepper.
Bring the sauce to a boil, reduce heat to medium-low, and simmer the sauce for 20 minutes.
Remove the sauce from the heat and stir in chopped basil.
Pour sauce over pasta and serve.
Servings: 4
Ready in Preparation Time: 35 minutes
Nutrition Facts
Percent daily values based on the Reference Daily Intake (RDI) for a 2000 calorie diet.
Nutrition:
Calories 564.35
Calories From Fat56.26
% Daily Value
Total Fat 6.44g
Saturated Fat 1.04g 5%
Cholesterol 0mg 0%
Sodium 766mg
Potassium 1448mg
Total Carbohydrates 102.47g
Fiber 17.64g
Sugar 11.83g
Protein 29g

Instant Savory Gigante Beans

Ingredients

1 lb Gigante Beans soaked overnight

1/2 cup olive oil

1 onion sliced

2 cloves garlic crushed or minced

1 red bell pepper (cut into 1/2-inch pieces)

2 carrots, sliced

1/2 tsp salt and ground black pepper

2 tomatoes peeled, grated

1 Tbsp celery (chopped)

1 Tbsp tomato paste (or ketchup)

3/4 tsp sweet paprika

1 tsp oregano

1 cup vegetable broth

Directions:

Soak Gigante beans overnight.

Press SAUTÉ button on your Instant Pot and heat the oil.

Sauté onion, garlic, sweet pepper, carrots with a pinch of salt for 3 - 4 minutes; stir occasionally.

Add rinsed Gigante beans into your Instant Pot along with all remaining ingredients and stir well.

Lock lid into place and set on the MANUAL setting for 25 minutes.

When the beep sounds, quick release the pressure by pressing Cancel, and twisting the steam handle to the Venting position.

Taste and adjust seasonings to taste.

Serve warm or cold.

Keep refrigerated.

Servings: 6

Ready in Preparation Time: 55 minutes

Nutrition Facts

Percent daily values based on the Reference Daily Intake (RDI) for a 2000 calorie diet.

Nutrition:

Calories 502.45

Calories From Fat173.16

% Daily Value

Total Fat 19.63g

Saturated Fat 2.86g

Cholesterol 0.41mg <1%
Sodium 326.4mg
Potassium 1869.29mg
Total Carbohydrates 63.17g
Fiber 15.63g
Sugar 6.37g
Protein 21.74g

Nettle Soup with Rice

Ingredients
3 Tbsp of olive oil
2 onions finely chopped
2 cloves garlic finely chopped
Salt and freshly ground black pepper
4 medium potatoes cut into cubes
1 cup of rice
1 Tbsp arrowroot
2 cups vegetable broth
2 cups of water
1 bunch of young nettle leaves packed
1/2 cup fresh parsley finely chopped
1 tsp cumin
Directions:
Heat olive oil in a large pot.
Sauté onion and garlic with a pinch of salt until softened.
Add potato, rice, and arrowroot; sauté for 2 to 3 minutes.
Pour broth and water, stir well, cover and cook over medium heat for about 20 minutes.
Cook over medium heat for about 20 minutes.
Add young nettle leaves, parsley, and cumin; stir and cook for 5 to 7 minutes.
Transfer the soup in a blender and blend until combined well.
Taste and adjust salt and pepper.
Serve hot.
Servings: 5
Ready in Preparation Time: 40 minutes
Nutrition Facts
Percent daily values based on the Reference Daily Intake (RDI) for a 2000 calorie diet.
Nutrition:
Calories 421.76
Calories From Fat88.32
% Daily Value
Total Fat 9.8g
Saturated Fat 1.54g 8%
Cholesterol 0.8mg <1%
Sodium 790.86mg
Potassium 963.6mg
Total Carbohydrates 73.52g
Fiber 8g
Sugar 3.3g
Protein 9.66g

Okra with Grated Tomatoes (Slow Cooker)

Ingredients
2 lbs fresh okra cleaned
2 onions finely chopped
2 cloves garlic finely sliced
2 carrots sliced
2 ripe tomatoes grated
1 cup of water
4 Tbsp olive oil
Salt and ground black pepper
1 Tbsp fresh parsley finely chopped
Directions:
Add okra in your Crock-Pot: sprinkle with a pinch of salt and pepper.
Add in chopped onion, garlic, carrots, and grated tomatoes; stir well.
Pour water and oil, season with the salt, pepper, and give a good stir.
Cover and cook on LOW for 2-3 hours or until tender.
Open the lid and add fresh parsley; stir.
Taste and adjust salt and pepper.
Serve hot.
Servings: 4
Ready in Preparation Time: 3 hours and 10 minutes
Nutrition Facts
Percent daily values based on the Reference Daily Intake (RDI) for a 2000 calorie diet.
Nutrition:
Calories 223.47
Calories From Fat123.5
% Daily Value
Total Fat 14g
Saturated Fat 1.96g
Cholesterol 0mg 0%
Sodium 51.91mg 2%
Potassium 1009.6mg
Total Carbohydrates 23.58g 8%
Fiber 9.47g
Sugar 6.62g
Protein 6g
Oven-baked Smoked Lentil 'Burgers'
Ingredients

1 1/2 cups dried lentils
3 cups of water
Salt and ground black pepper to taste
2 Tbsp olive oil
1 onion finely diced
2 cloves minced garlic
1 cup button mushrooms sliced
2 Tbsp tomato paste
1/2 tsp fresh basil finely chopped
1 cup chopped almonds
3 tsp balsamic vinegar
3 Tbsp coconut aminos
1 tsp liquid smoke
3/4 cup silken tofu soft
3/4 cup corn starch
Directions:
Cook lentils in salted water until tender or for about 30-35 minutes; rinse, drain, and set aside.
Heat oil in a frying skillet and sauté onion, garlic and mushrooms for 4 to 5 minutes; stir occasionally.
Stir in the tomato paste, salt, basil, salt, and black pepper; cook for 2 to 3 minutes.
Stir in almonds, vinegar, coconut aminos, liquid smoke, and lentils.
Remove from heat and stir in blended tofu and corn starch.
Keep stirring until all ingredients combined well.
Form mixture into patties and refrigerate for an hour.
Preheat oven to 350 F.
Line a baking dish with parchment paper and arrange patties on the pan.
1Bake for 20 to 25 minutes.
1Serve hot with buns, green salad, tomato sauce...etc.
Servings: 6
Ready in Preparation Time: 1 hour and 20 minutes
Nutrition Facts
Percent daily values based on the Reference Daily Intake (RDI) for a 2000 calorie diet.
Nutrition:
Calories 439.12
Calories From Fat148.97
% Daily Value
Total Fat 17.48g
Saturated Fat 1.71g 9%

Cholesterol 0mg 0%
Sodium 330mg
Potassium 805.8mg
Total Carbohydrates 53.72g
Fiber 18.19g
Sugar 4.6g
Protein 19.37g

Powerful Spinach and Mustard Leaves Puree

Ingredients
2 Tbsp almond butter
1 onion finely diced
2 Tbsp minced garlic
1 tsp salt and black pepper (or to taste)
1 lb mustard leaves, cleaned rinsed
1 lb frozen spinach thawed
1 tsp coriander
1 tsp ground cumin
1/2 cup almond milk
Directions:
Press the SAUTÉ button on your Instant Pot and heat the almond butter.
Sauté onion, garlic, and a pinch of salt for 2-3 minutes; stir occasionally.
Add spinach and the mustard greens and stir for a minute or two.
Season with the salt and pepper, coriander, and cumin; give a good stir.
Lock lid into place and set on the MANUAL setting for 15 minutes.
Use Quick Release - turn the valve from sealing to venting to release the pressure.
Transfer mixture to a blender, add almond milk and blend until smooth.
Taste and adjust seasonings.
Serve.
Servings: 4
Ready in Preparation Time: 50 minutes
Nutrition Facts
Percent daily values based on the Reference Daily Intake (RDI) for a 2000 calorie diet.
Nutrition:
Calories 180.53
Calories From Fat82.69
% Daily Value
Total Fat 10g
Saturated Fat 0.65g 3%
Cholesterol 0mg 0%
Sodium 1519.12mg
Potassium 846mg
Total Carbohydrates 17.46g 6%
Fiber 6.92g
Sugar 2.13g
Protein 10.65g

Quinoa and Rice Stuffed Peppers (oven-baked)

Ingredients
3/4 cup long-grain rice
8 bell peppers (any color)
2 Tbsp olive oil
1 onion finely diced
2 cloves chopped garlic
1 can (11 oz) crushed tomatoes
1 tsp cumin
1 tsp coriander
4 Tbsp ground walnuts
2 cups cooked quinoa
4 Tbsp chopped parsley
Salt and ground black pepper to taste
Directions:
Preheat oven to 400 F/200 C.
Boil rice and drain in a colander.
Cut the top stem section of the pepper off, remove the remaining pith and seeds, rinse peppers.
Heat oil in a large frying skillet, and sauté onion and garlic until soft.
Add tomatoes, cumin, ground almonds, salt, pepper, and coriander; stir well and simmer for 2 minutes stirring constantly.
Remove from the heat and add the rice, quinoa, and parsley; stir well.
Taste and adjust salt and pepper.
Fill the peppers with a mixture, and place peppers cut side-up in a baking dish; drizzle with little oil.
Bake for 15 minutes.
1Serve warm.
Servings: 8
Ready in Preparation Time: 35 minutes
Nutrition Facts
Percent daily values based on the Reference Daily Intake (RDI) for a 2000 calorie diet.
Nutrition:
Calories 335.69
Calories From Fat83.63
% Daily Value
Total Fat 9.58g
Saturated Fat 1.2g 5%

Cholesterol 0mg 0%
Sodium 66.14mg 3%
Potassium 678.73mg
Total Carbohydrates 55.13g
Fiber 8.25g
Sugar 7.8g
Protein 9.8g

Quinoa and Lentils with Crushed Tomato

Ingredients
4 Tbsp olive oil
1 medium onion, diced
2 garlic clove, minced
Salt and ground black pepper to taste
1 can (15 oz) tomatoes crushed
1 cup vegetable broth
1/2 cup quinoa, washed and drained
1 cup cooked lentils
1 tsp chili powder
1 tsp cumin
Directions:
Heat oil in a pot and sauté the onion and garlic with the pinch of salt until soft.
Pour reserved tomatoes and vegetable broth, bring to boil, and stir well.
Stir in the quinoa, cover and cook for 15 minutes; stir occasionally.
Add in lentils, chili powder, and cumin; cook for further 5 minutes.
Taste and adjust seasonings.
Serve immediately.
Keep refrigerated in a covered container for 4 - 5 days.
Servings: 4
Ready in Preparation Time: 35 minutes
Nutrition Facts
Percent daily values based on the Reference Daily Intake (RDI) for a 2000 calorie diet.
Nutrition:
Calories 397.45
Calories From Fat138.18
% Daily Value
Total Fat 15.61g
Saturated Fat 2.14g
Cholesterol 0mg 0%
Sodium 343.8mg
Potassium 738.51mg
Total Carbohydrates 49.32g
Fiber 16.7g
Sugar 2.35g
Protein 16.6g

Silk Tofu Penne with Spinach

Ingredients

1 lb penne, uncooked
12 oz of frozen spinach, thawed
1 cup silken tofu mashed
1/2 cup soy milk (unsweetened)
1/2 cup vegetable broth
1 Tbsp white wine vinegar
1/2 tsp Italian seasoning
Salt and ground pepper to taste

Directions:

Cook penne pasta according to package directions; rinse and drain in a colander.
Drain spinach well, squeezing out excess liquid.
Place spinach with all remaining ingredients in a blender and beat until smooth.
Pour the spinach mixture over pasta.
Taste and adjust the salt and pepper.
Store pasta in an airtight container in the refrigerator for 3 to 5 days.
Servings: 4
Ready in Preparation Time: 25 minutes
Nutrition Facts
Percent daily values based on the Reference Daily Intake (RDI) for a 2000 calorie diet.
Nutrition:
Calories 492.8
Calories From Fat (5%) 27.06
% Daily Value
Total Fat 3.07g 5%
Saturated Fat 0.38g 2%
Cholesterol 0.31mg <1%
Sodium 491.22mg
Potassium 433mg
Total Carbohydrates 92.45g
Fiber 7.8g
Sugar 1.21g
Protein 21.61g

Slow-Cooked Butter Beans, Okra and Potatoes Stew

Ingredients

2 cups frozen butter (lima) beans, thawed

1 cup frozen okra, thawed

2 large Russet potatoes cut into cubes

1 can (6 oz) whole-kernel corn, drained

1 large carrot sliced

1 green bell pepper finely chopped

1 cup green peas

1/2 cup chopped celery

1 medium onion finely chopped

2 cups vegetable broth

2 cans (6 oz) tomato sauce

1 cup of water

1/2 tsp salt and freshly ground black pepper

Directions:

Combine all ingredients in your Slow Cooker; give a good stir.

Cover and cook on HIGH for 6 hours.

Taste, adjust seasonings, and serve hot.

Servings: 6

Ready in Preparation Time: 6 hours and 5 minutes

Nutrition Facts

Percent daily values based on the Reference Daily Intake (RDI) for a 2000 calorie diet.

Nutrition:

Calories 241.71

Calories From Fat (5%) 11.22

% Daily Value

Total Fat 1.28g 2%

Saturated Fat 0.27g 1%

Cholesterol 0mg 0%

Sodium 714.16mg

Potassium 1228mg

Total Carbohydrates 49.6g

Fiber 9.65g

Sugar 8.17g

Protein 10.57g

Soya Minced Stuffed Eggplants

Ingredients

2 eggplants
1/3 cup sesame oil
1 onion finely chopped
2 garlic cloves minced
1 lb soya mince* see note
Salt and ground black pepper
1/3 cup almond milk
2 Tbsp fresh parsley, chopped
1/3 cup fresh basil chopped
1 tsp fennel powder
1 cup of water
4 Tbsp tomato paste (fresh or canned)

Directions:

Rinse and slice the eggplant in half lengthwise.
Submerge sliced eggplant into a container with salted water.
Soak soya mince in water for 10 to 15 minutes.
Preheat oven to 400 F.
Rinse eggplant and dry with a clean towel.
Heat oil in large frying skillet, and sauté onion and garlic with a pinch of salt until softened.
Add drained soya mince, and cook over medium heat until cooked through.
Add all remaining ingredients (except water and tomato paste) and cook for a further 5 minutes; remove from heat.
Scoop out the seed part of each eggplant.
1Spoon in the filling and arrange stuffed eggplants onto the large baking dish.
1Dissolve tomato paste into the water and pour evenly over eggplants.
1Bake for 20 to 25 minutes.
1Serve warm.
Servings: 4
Ready in Preparation Time: 1 hour
Nutrition Facts
Percent daily values based on the Reference Daily Intake (RDI) for a 2000 calorie diet.
Nutrition:
Calories 287.32
Calories From Fat141.77
% Daily Value

Total Fat 16.42g
Saturated Fat 2.02g
Cholesterol 0mg 0%
Sodium 104.72mg 4%
Potassium 1150.5mg
Total Carbohydrates 24.67g 8%
Fiber 11.16g
Sugar 4.75g
Protein 16.16g

Triple Beans and Corn Salad

Ingredients
1 can (15 oz) kidney beans, drained and rinsed
1 can (15 oz) white beans, drained and rinsed
1 can (15 oz) black beans, rinsed and drained
1 can (11 oz) frozen corn kernels thawed
1 green bell pepper, chopped
1 red onion, chopped
1 clove crushed garlic
1 Tbsp salt and ground black pepper to taste
1/2 cup olive oil
3 Tbsp red wine vinegar
3 Tbsp lemon juice
1/4 cup chopped fresh cilantro
1/2 Tbsp ground cumin
Directions:
In a large bowl, combine beans, corn, pepper, onion, and garlic.
Season salad with the salt and pepper; stir to combine well.
In a separate bowl, whisk together olive oil, red wine vinegar, lemon juice, cilantro, and cumin.
Pour olive oil dressing over salad, and toss to combine well.
Refrigerate for one hour and serve.
Servings: 8
Ready in Preparation Time: 15 minutes
Nutrition Facts
Percent daily values based on the Reference Daily Intake (RDI) for a 2000 calorie diet.
Nutrition:
Calories 696
Calories From Fat155.25
% Daily Value
Total Fat 17.62g
Saturated Fat 3g
Cholesterol 0mg 0%
Sodium 1118mg
Potassium 1719.68mg
Total Carbohydrates 102.9g
Fiber 25g 102%
Sugar 1.68g
Protein 36.94g

Vegan Raw Pistachio Flaxseed 'Burgers'

Ingredients
1 cup ground flaxseed
1 cup pistachio finely sliced
2 cups cooked spinach drained
2 Tbsp sesame oil
4 cloves garlic finely sliced
2 Tbsp lemon juice, freshly squeezed
Sea salt to taste
Directions:
Add all ingredients into a food processor or high-speed blender; process until combined well.
Form mixture into patties.
Refrigerate for one hour.
Serve with your favorite vegetable dip.
Servings: 4
Ready in Preparation Time: 15 minutes
Nutrition Facts
Percent daily values based on the Reference Daily Intake (RDI) for a 2000 calorie diet.
Nutrition:
Calories 273
Calories From Fat184.41
% Daily Value
Total Fat 21.6g
Saturated Fat 2.72g
Cholesterol 0mg 0%
Sodium 322.9mg
Potassium 637mg
Total Carbohydrates 14.8g 5%
Fiber 7g
Sugar 3.1g
Protein 10.46g

Chapter 6. Dessert And Snack Recipes

Banana-Nut Bread Bars

Preparation Time: 5 minutes
Cooking Time: 30 minutes
Servings: 9 bars
Ingredients
Nonstick cooking spray (optional)
2 large ripe bananas
1 tablespoon maple syrup
½ Teaspoon vanilla extract
2 cups old-fashioned rolled oats
½ Teaspoons salt
¼ Cup chopped walnuts
Directions:
Preheat the oven to 350°f. Lightly coat a 9-by-9-inch baking pan with nonstick cooking spray (if using) or line with parchment paper for oil-free baking.
In a medium bowl, mash the bananas with a fork. Add the maple syrup and vanilla extract and mix well. Add the oats, salt, and walnuts, mixing well.
Transfer the batter to the baking pan and bake for 25 to 30 minutes, until the top is crispy. Cool completely before slicing into 9 bars. Transfer to an airtight storage container or a large plastic bag.
Nutrition (1 bar): calories: 73; fat: 1g; protein: 2g; carbohydrates: 15g; fiber: 2g; sugar: 5g; sodium: 129mg

Lemon Coconut Cilantro Rolls

Preparation Time: 30 minutes • chill Preparation Time: 30 minutes
Servings: 16 pieces
Ingredients

½ Cup fresh cilantro, chopped
1 cup sprouts (clover, alfalfa)
1 garlic clove, pressed
2 tablespoons ground brazil nuts or almonds
2 tablespoons flaked coconut
1 tablespoon coconut oil
Pinch cayenne pepper
Pinch sea salt
Pinch freshly ground black pepper
Zest and juice of 1 lemon
2 tablespoons ground flaxseed
1 to 2 tablespoons water
2 whole-wheat wraps, or corn wraps

Directions:
Put everything but the wraps in a food processor and pulse to combine. Or combine the Ingredients in a large bowl. Add the water, if needed, to help the mix come together.
Spread the mixture out over each wrap, roll it up, and place it in the fridge for 30 minutes to set.
Remove the rolls from the fridge and slice each into 8 pieces to serve as appetizers or sides with a soup or stew.
Get the best flavor by buying whole raw brazil nuts or almonds, toasting them lightly in a dry skillet or toaster oven, and then grinding them in a coffee grinder.
Nutrition (1 piece) calories: 66; total fat: 4g; carbs: 6g; fiber: 1g; protein: 2g

Tamari Almonds

Preparation Time: 5 minutes
Cooking Time: 15 minutes
Servings: 8
Ingredients

1 pound raw almonds
3 tablespoons tamari or soy sauce
2 tablespoons extra-virgin olive oil
1 tablespoon Nutritional yeast
1 to 2 teaspoons chili powder, to taste

Directions:
Preheat the oven to 400°f.
Line a baking sheet with parchment paper.
In a medium bowl, combine the almonds, tamari, and olive oil until well coated.
Spread the almonds on the prepared baking sheet and roast for 10 to 15 minutes, until browned.
Cool for 10 minutes, then season with the Nutritional yeast and chili powder.
Transfer to a glass jar and close tightly with a lid.
Nutrition: calories: 364; fat: 32g; protein: 13g; carbohydrates: 13g; fiber: 7g; sugar: 3g; sodium: 381mg

Tempeh Taco Bites

Preparation Time: 5 minutes
Cooking Time: 45 minutes
Servings: 3 dozen
Ingredients

8 ounces tempeh
3 tablespoons soy sauce
2 teaspoons ground cumin
1 teaspoon chili powder
1 teaspoon dried oregano
1 tablespoon olive oil
1/2 cup finely minced onion
2 garlic cloves, minced
Salt and freshly ground black pepper
2 tablespoons tomato paste
1 chipotle chile in adobo, finely minced
1/4 cup hot water or vegetable broth, homemade or store-bought, plus more if needed
36 phyllo pastry cups, thawed
1/2 cup basic guacamole, homemade or store-bought
18 ripe cherry tomatoes, halved

Directions
In a medium saucepan of simmering water, cook the tempeh for 30 minutes. Drain well, then finely mince and place it in a bowl. Add the soy sauce, cumin, chili powder, and oregano. Mix well and set aside.
In a medium skillet, heat the oil over medium heat. Add the onion, cover, and cook for 5 minutes. Stir in the garlic, then add the tempeh mixture and cook, stirring, for 2 to 3 minutes. Season with salt and pepper to taste. Set aside.
In a small bowl, combine the tomato paste, chipotle, and the hot water or broth. Return tempeh mixture to heat and in stir tomato-chile mixture and cook for 10 to 15 minutes, stirring occasionally, until the liquid is absorbed.
The mixture should be fairly dry, but if it begins to stick to the pan, add a little more hot water, 1 tablespoon at a time. Taste, adjusting seasonings if necessary. Remove from the heat.
To assemble, fill the phyllo cups to the top with the tempeh filling, using about 2 teaspoons of filling in each. Top with a dollop of guacamole and a cherry tomato half and serve.

Mushroom Croustades

Preparation Time: 10 minutes
Cooking Time: 10 minutes
Servings: 12 croustades
Ingredients

12 thin slices whole-grain bread
1 tablespoon olive oil, plus more for brushing bread
2 medium shallots, chopped
2 garlic cloves, minced
12 ounces white mushrooms, chopped
¼ cup chopped fresh parsley
1 teaspoon dried thyme
1 tablespoon soy sauce

Directions
Preheat the oven to 400°f. Using a 3-inch round pastry cutter or a drinking glass, cut a circle from each bread slice. Brush the bread circles with oil and press them firmly but gently into a mini-muffin tin. Bake until the bread is toasted, about 10 minutes.
Meanwhile, in a large skillet, heat the 1 tablespoon oil over medium heat. Add the shallots, garlic, and mushrooms and sauté for 5 minutes to soften the vegetables. Stir in the parsley, thyme, and soy sauce and cook until the liquid is absorbed, about 5 minutes longer. Spoon the mushroom mixture into the croustade cups and return to the oven for 3 to 5 minutes to heat through. Serve warm.

Stuffed Cherry Tomatoes

Preparation Time: 15 minutes
Cooking Time: 0 minutes
Servings: 6
Ingredients

2 pints cherry tomatoes, tops removed and centers scooped out
2 avocados, mashed
Juice of 1 lemon
½ Red bell pepper, minced
4 green onions (white and green parts), finely minced
1 tablespoon minced fresh tarragon
Pinch of sea salt

Directions:
Place the cherry tomatoes open-side up on a platter.
In a small bowl, -combine the avocado, lemon juice, bell pepper, scallions, tarragon, and salt.
Stir until well -combined. Scoop into the cherry tomatoes and serve immediately.

Spicy Black Bean Dip

Preparation Time: 10 minutes
Cooking Time: 0 minutes
Servings: 2 cups
Ingredients
1 (14-ounce) can black beans, drained and rinsed, or 1½ cups cooked
Zest and juice of 1 lime
1 tablespoon tamari, or soy sauce
¼ Cup water
¼ Cup fresh cilantro, chopped
1 teaspoon ground cumin
Pinch cayenne pepper

Directions:
Put the beans in a food processor (best choice) or blender, along with the lime zest and juice, tamari, and about ¼ cup of water.
Blend until smooth, then blend in the cilantro, cumin, and cayenne.
If you don't have a blender or prefer a different consistency, simply transfer it to a bowl once the beans have been puréed and stir in the spices, instead of forcing the blender.
Nutrition (1 cup) calories: 190; total fat: 1g; carbs: 35g; fiber: 12g; protein: 13g

Cheezy Cashew–Roasted Red Pepper Toasts

Preparation Time: 15 minutes
Cooking Time: 0 minutes
Servings: 16 to 24 toasts
Ingredients

2 jarred roasted red peppers
1 cup unsalted cashews
¼ cup water
1 tablespoon soy sauce
2 tablespoons chopped green onions
¼ cup Nutritional yeast
2 tablespoons balsamic vinegar
2 tablespoons olive oil

Directions
Use canapé or cookie cutters to cut the bread into desired shapes about 2 inches wide. If you don't have a cutter, use a knife to cut the bread into squares, triangles, or rectangles. You should get 2 to 4 pieces out of each slice of bread. Toast the bread and set aside to cool.
Coarsely chop 1 red pepper and set aside. Cut the remaining pepper into thin strips or decorative shapes and set aside for garnish.
In a blender or food processor, grind the cashews to a fine powder. Add the water and soy sauce and process until smooth. Add the chopped red pepper and puree. Add the green onions, Nutritional yeast, vinegar, and oil and process until smooth and well blended.
Spread a spoonful of the pepper mixture onto each of the toasted bread pieces and top decoratively with the reserved pepper strips. Arrange on a platter or tray and serve.

Baked Potato Chips

Preparation Time: 10 minutes
Cooking Time: 30 minutes
Servings: 4
Ingredients

1 large russet potato
1 teaspoon paprika
½ Teaspoon garlic salt
¼ Teaspoon vegan sugar
¼ Teaspoon onion powder
¼ Teaspoon chipotle powder or chili powder
⅛ Teaspoon salt
⅛ Teaspoon ground mustard
⅛ Teaspoon ground cayenne pepper
1 teaspoon canola oil
⅛ Teaspoon liquid smoke

Directions:
Wash and peel the potato. Cut into thin, 1/10-inch slices (a mandoline slicer or the slicer blade in a food processor is helpful for consistently sized slices).
Fill a large bowl with enough very cold water to cover the potato. Transfer the potato slices to the bowl and soak for 20 minutes.
Preheat the oven to 400°f. Line a baking sheet with parchment paper.
In a small bowl, combine the paprika, garlic salt, sugar, onion powder, chipotle powder, salt, mustard, and cayenne.
Drain and rinse the potato slices and pat dry with a paper towel.
Transfer to a large bowl.
Add the canola oil, liquid smoke, and spice mixture to the bowl. Toss to coat.
Transfer the potatoes to the prepared baking sheet.
Bake for 15 minutes. Flip the chips over and bake for 15 minutes longer, until browned.
Transfer the chips to 4 storage containers or large glass jars.
Let cool before closing the lids tightly.
Nutrition: calories: 89; fat: 1g; protein: 2g; carbohydrates: 18g; fiber: 2g; sugar: 1g; sodium: 65mg

Mushrooms Stuffed With Spinach And Walnuts

Preparation Time: 10 minutes
Cooking Time: 6 minutes
Servings: 4 to 6 servings
Ingredients
2 tablespoons olive oil
8 ounces white mushroom, lightly rinsed, patted dry, and stems reserved
1 garlic clove, minced
1 cup cooked spinach
1 cup finely chopped walnuts
1/2 cup unseasoned dry bread crumbs
Salt and freshly ground black pepper
Directions
Preheat the oven to 400°f. Lightly oil a large baking pan and set aside. In a large skillet, heat the oil over medium heat. Add the mushroom caps and cook for 2 minutes to soften slightly. Remove from the skillet and set aside.
Chop the mushroom stems and add to the same skillet. Add the garlic and cook over medium heat until softened, about 2 minutes. Stir in the spinach, walnuts, bread crumbs, and salt and pepper to taste. Cook for 2 minutes, stirring well to combine.
Fill the reserved mushroom caps with the stuffing mixture and arrange in the baking pan. Bake until the mushrooms are tender and the filling is hot, about 10 minutes. Serve hot.

Salsa Fresca

Preparation Time: 15 minutes
Cooking Time: 0 minutes
Servings: 4
Ingredients
3 large heirloom tomatoes or other fresh tomatoes, chopped
½ Red onion, finely chopped
½ Bunch cilantro, chopped
2 garlic cloves, minced
1 jalapeño, minced
Juice of 1 lime, or 1 tablespoon prepared lime juice
¼ Cup olive oil
Sea salt
Whole-grain tortilla chips, for serving
Directions:
In a small bowl, combine the tomatoes, onion, cilantro, garlic, jalapeño, lime juice, and olive oil and mix well. Allow to sit at room temperature for 15 minutes. Season with salt. Serve with tortilla chips.
The salsa can be stored in an airtight container in the refrigerator for up to 1 week.

6 Guacamole
Preparation Time: 10 minutes
Cooking Time: 0 minutes
Servings: 2
Ingredients
2 ripe avocados
2 garlic cloves, pressed
Zest and juice of 1 lime
1 teaspoon ground cumin
Pinch sea salt
Pinch freshly ground black pepper
Pinch cayenne pepper (optional)
Directions:
Mash the avocados in a large bowl. Add the rest of the Ingredients and stir to combine.
Try adding diced tomatoes (cherry are divine), chopped scallions or chives, chopped fresh cilantro or basil, lemon rather than lime, paprika, or whatever you think would taste good!
Nutrition (1 cup) calories: 258; total fat: 22g; carbs: 18g; fiber: 11g; protein: 4g

Veggie Hummus Pinwheels

Preparation Time: 10 minutes
Cooking Time: 0 minutes
Servings: 3
Ingredients

3 whole-grain, spinach, flour, or gluten-free tortillas
3 large swiss chard leaves
¾ Cup edamame hummus or prepared hummus
¾ Cup shredded carrots

Directions:
Lay 1 tortilla flat on a cutting board.
Place 1 swiss chard leaf over the tortilla. Spread ¼ cup of hummus over the swiss chard.
Spread ¼ cup of carrots over the hummus. Starting at one end of the tortilla, roll tightly toward the opposite side.
Slice each roll up into 6 pieces. Place in a single-serving storage container.
Repeat with the remaining tortillas and filling and seal the lids.
Nutrition: calories: 254; fat: 8g; protein: 10g; carbohydrates: 39g; fiber: 8g; sugar: 4g; sodium: 488mg

Asian Lettuce Rolls

Preparation Time: 15 minutes
Cooking Time: 5 minutes
Servings: 4
Ingredients
2 ounces rice noodles
2 tablespoons chopped thai basil
2 tablespoons chopped cilantro
1 garlic clove, minced
1 tablespoon minced fresh ginger
Juice of ½ lime, or 2 teaspoons prepared lime juice
2 tablespoons soy sauce
1 cucumber, julienned
2 carrots, peeled and julienned
8 leaves butter lettuce
Directions:
Cook the rice noodles according to package Directions.
In a small bowl, whisk together the basil, cilantro, garlic, ginger, lime juice, and soy sauce.
Toss with the cooked noodles, cucumber, and carrots.
Divide the mixture evenly among lettuce leaves and roll.
Secure with a toothpick and serve immediately.

Pinto-Pecan Fireballs

Preparation Time: 5 minutes
Cooking Time: 30 minutes
Servings: about 20 pieces
Ingredients

1-1⁄2 cups cooked or 1 (15.5-ounce) can pinto beans, drained and rinsed
1⁄2 cup chopped pecans
1⁄4 cup minced green onions
1 garlic clove, minced
3 tablespoons wheat gluten flour (vital wheat gluten)
3 tablespoons unseasoned dry bread crumbs
4 tablespoons tabasco or other hot sauce
1⁄4 teaspoon salt
1⁄8 teaspoon ground cayenne
1⁄4 cup vegan margarine

Directions
Preheat the oven to 350°f. Lightly oil a 9 x 13-inch baking pan and set aside. Blot the drained beans well with a paper towel, pressing out any excess liquid. In a food processor, combine the pinto beans, pecans, green onions, garlic, flour, bread crumbs, 2 tablespoons of the tabasco, salt, and cayenne. Pulse until well combined, leaving some texture. Use your hands to roll the mixture firmly into 1-inch balls.
Place the balls in the prepared baking pan and bake until nicely browned, about 25 to 30 minutes, turning halfway through.
Meanwhile, in small saucepan, combine the remaining 2 tablespoons tabasco and the margarine and melt over low heat. Pour the sauce over the fireballs and bake 10 minutes longer. Serve immediately.

Sweet Potato Biscuits

Preparation Time: 60 minutes
Cooking Time: 10 minutes
Servings: 12 biscuits
Ingredients
1 medium sweet potato
3 tablespoons melted coconut oil, divided
1 tablespoon maple syrup
1 cup whole-wheat flour
2 teaspoons baking powder
Pinch sea salt
Directions:
Bake the sweet potato at 350°F for about 45 minutes, until tender.
Allow it to cool, then remove the flesh and mash.
Turn the oven up to 375°F and line a baking sheet with parchment paper or lightly grease it. Measure out 1 cup potato flesh.
In a medium bowl, combine the mashed sweet potato with 1½ tablespoons of the coconut oil and the maple syrup. Mix together the flour and baking powder in a separate medium bowl, then add the flour mixture to the potato mixture and blend well with a fork.
Put the rounds onto the prepared baking sheet. Brush the top of each with some of the remaining 1½ tablespoons melted coconut oil. Bake 10 minutes, or until lightly golden on top. Serve hot.
Nutrition (1 biscuit) calories: 116; total fat: 4g; carbs: 19g; fiber: 3g; protein: 3g

Lemon And Garlic Marinated Mushrooms

Preparation Time: 15 minutes
Cooking Time: 0 minutes
Servings: 4 servings
Ingredients

3 tablespoons olive oil
2 tablespoons fresh lemon juice
2 garlic cloves, crushed
1 teaspoon dried marjoram
1/2 teaspoon coarsely ground fennel seed
1/2 teaspoon salt
1/4 teaspoon freshly ground black pepper
8 ounces small white mushrooms, lightly rinsed, patted dry, and stemmed
1 tablespoon minced fresh parsley

Directions
In a medium bowl, whisk together the oil, lemon juice, garlic, marjoram, fennel seed, salt, and pepper. Add the mushrooms and parsley and stir gently until coated.
Cover and refrigerate for at least 2 hours or overnight. Stir well before serving.

Garlic Toast

Preparation Time: 5 minutes
Cooking Time: 5 minutes
Servings: 1 slice
Ingredients

1 teaspoon coconut oil, or olive oil
Pinch sea salt
1 to 2 teaspoons Nutritional yeast
1 small garlic clove, pressed, or ¼ teaspoon garlic powder
1 slice whole-grain bread

Directions:
In a small bowl, mix together the oil, salt, Nutritional yeast, and garlic.
You can either toast the bread and then spread it with the seasoned oil, or brush the oil on the bread and put it in a toaster oven to bake for 5 minutes.
If you're using fresh garlic, it's best to spread it onto the bread and then bake it.
Nutrition (1 slice) calories: 138; total fat: 6g; carbs: 16g; fiber: 4g; protein: 7g

Chapter 7. Vegetables

Peanut Slaw with Soba Noodles

Preparation Time: 40 minutes
Cooking Time: 0 minute
Servings: 4
Ingredients:
For the Slaw:
½ pound Brussels sprouts
1 bunch of green onions, sliced into thin rounds
6 cups shredded green cabbage
4 medium carrots, grated
4 ounces soba noodles, cooked
For the Peanut Dressing:
1 teaspoon minced garlic
1 tablespoon grated ginger
2 tablespoons honey
3 tablespoons rice vinegar
3 tablespoons soy sauce
½ cup peanut butter
3 tablespoons toasted sesame oil
For the Garnish:
¼ cup chopped cilantro
2 tablespoons chopped peanuts
1 lime, sliced into wedges
Directions:
Prepare the dressing and for this, place all its ingredients in a large bowl and whisk until smooth.
Place noodles in a large bowl, add all the vegetables, pour in the prepared dressing and toss until well coated.
Let the slaw marinate for 30 minutes, top with peanuts and cilantro and serve with lime wedges.
Nutrition:
Calories: 265 Cal
Fat: 14 g
Carbs: 31.2 g
Protein: 9 g,
Fiber: 4.6 g

Thai Green Curry with Spring Vegetables

Preparation Time: 10 minutes
Cooking Time: 35 minutes
Servings: 4
Ingredients:
2 cups sliced asparagus
1 small white onion, peeled, diced
2 cups baby spinach, chopped
1 cup sliced carrots
1 teaspoon minced garlic
1 tablespoon chopped ginger
1 cup brown rice, cooked
2 tablespoons Thai green curry paste
1 ½ teaspoon coconut sugar
1/8 teaspoon salt
1 ½ teaspoon lime juice
2 teaspoons olive oil
1 ½ teaspoons soy sauce
14 ounces coconut milk, unsweetened
½ cup of water
Directions:
Take a large skillet pan, place it over medium heat, add oil and when hot, add ginger, onion, and garlic and cook for 5 minutes.
Then add carrots and asparagus, cook for 3 minutes, stir in curry paste and continue cooking for 2 minutes.
Pour in milk and water, stir in sugar and bring the curry to simmer.
Switch heat to the low level, simmer for 10 minutes until cooked, then stir in spinach and cook for 30 seconds until spinach leaves wilt.
When done, remove the pan from heat, stir in lime juice and soy sauce, taste to adjust seasoning and garnish with cilantro.
Serve curry with boiled rice.
Nutrition:
Calories: 400 Cal
Fat: 22.1 g
Carbs: 49 g
Protein: 8.6 g
Fiber: 6.1 g

Mango Cabbage Wraps

Preparation Time: 15 minutes
Cooking Time: 35 minutes
Servings: 4
Ingredients:
2 tablespoons chopped peanuts, toasted
1 small head of green cabbage
2 tablespoons coconut flakes, unsweetened, toasted
For the Baked Tofu:
15 ounces tofu, extra-firm, drained, cut into ½-inch cubed
2 teaspoons cornstarch
1 tablespoon soy sauce
1 tablespoon olive oil
For the Peanut Sauce:
1 teaspoon minced garlic
2 tablespoons soy sauce
2 tablespoons apple cider vinegar
4 tablespoons lime juice
2 tablespoons honey
1/3 cup peanut butter
2 teaspoons toasted sesame oil
For the Mango Pico:
4 green onions, chopped
2 mangos, peeled, stoned, diced
1 medium red bell pepper, cored, chopped
1 jalapeño, minced
1/3 cup cilantro leaves, chopped
¼ teaspoon salt
2 tablespoons lime juice
Directions:
Prepare tofu and for this, place tofu pieces on a baking sheet, drizzle with 1 tablespoon oil and soy sauce, and toss until coated.

Sprinkle with 1 teaspoon cornstarch, toss until incorporated, sprinkle with remaining corn starch, toss until well coated, arrange tofu pieces in a single layer and bake for 35 minutes at 400 degrees F until crispy and golden brown.

Meanwhile, prepare the peanut sauce and for this, place all its ingredients in a food processor and pulse for 2 minutes until blended, set aside until required.

Prepare the salsa and for this, place all its ingredients in a bowl and toss until mixed.

When tofu has baked, take a pan, place it over medium heat, add toast peanuts and coconut flakes in it, and then add tofu pieces.

Pour in two-third of the peanut sauce, toss until well coated, cook for 5 minutes until its edges begin to bowl, then transfer tofu to a plate and let cool for 10 minutes.

Prepare the wrap and for this, pull out one leaf at a time from the cabbage, add some salsa, top with tofu, drizzle with remaining peanut sauce and serve.

Nutrition:

Calories: 448 Cal

Fat: 26 g

Carbs: 40 g

Protein: 20 g

Fiber: 6.6 g

Zucchanoush

Preparation Time: 10 minutes
Cooking Time: 10 minutes
Servings: 7
Ingredients:
1 pound small zucchini, quartered lengthwise
3 tablespoons mint leaves, divided
½ teaspoon minced garlic
1/3 teaspoon ground black pepper
2/3 teaspoon salt
2 tablespoons lemon juice
3 tablespoons olive oil, divided
1/4 cup tahini
1 tablespoon pine nuts, toasted
Directions:
Place zucchini pieces in a bowl, add 1 tablespoon oil, season with ½ teaspoon salt, toss until well coated, and then grill for 10 minutes over medium heat until evenly charred. Then transfer grilled zucchini to a food processor, add remaining ingredients, except for mint and nuts, and process for 2 minutes until blended.
Tip the mixture in a bowl, garnish with mint and nuts and then serve.
Nutrition:
Calories: 125 Cal
Fat: 11.5 g
Carbs: 4.5 g
Protein: 3 g
Fiber: 1 g

Grilled Asparagus and Shiitake Tacos

Preparation Time: 5 minutes
Cooking Time: 15 minutes
Servings: 4
Ingredients:
8 ounces shiitake mushrooms, destemmed
1 bunch of green onions
2 teaspoons minced garlic
1 teaspoon ground chipotle chili
1/2 teaspoon salt
3 tablespoons olive oil
8 corn tortillas, warmed
4 lime wedges
1 cup guacamole
¼ cup cilantro sprigs
4 tablespoons hot sauce
Directions:
Take a large baking dish, add garlic, salt, and chipotle and stir in oil until combined.
Add all the vegetables, toss until well coated, and then grill over medium heat until lightly charred, 6 minutes grilling time for asparagus, 5 minutes for onions and mushrooms.
When done, cut vegetables for 2-inch pieces, distribute them evenly between tortillas, top with cilantro, guacamole, and hot sauce and serve with lime wedges.
Nutrition:
Calories: 350 Cal
Fat: 21 g
Carbs: 36 g
Protein: 7 g
Fiber: 11 g

Mushroom and Quinoa Burger

Preparation Time: 15 minutes
Cooking Time: 40 minutes
Servings: 5
Ingredients:
For the Burgers:
1 cup cooked quinoa
4 medium caps of Portobello mushroom, gills removed, chopped
1/4 cup chopped red onion
½ teaspoon minced garlic
3 green onions, chopped
1/2 cup cornstarch
1/2 cup walnuts
2 teaspoons rice wine vinegar
2 tablespoons olive oil
5 whole-grain burger buns
For Toppings:
Sprouts as needed
Lettuce as needed
Sliced tomatoes as needed
Vegan mayonnaise as needed
Directions:
Prepare the burgers and for this, place mushrooms in a baking dish, add garlic and nuts, drizzle with 1 tablespoon oil, season with ¾ teaspoon salt and ¼ teaspoon black pepper, and then bake for 20 minutes until tender.
Then transfer the mushroom mixture in a food processor, add remaining ingredients for a burger, except for buns, stir until well mixed and then shape the mixture into five patties.
Fry the patties in batches for 5 minutes until browned and then bake for 10 minutes at 375 degrees F until thoroughly cooked.
Sandwich patties in burger buns, top with mayonnaise, sprouts, lettuce and tomatoes, and then serve.
Nutrition:
Calories: 495 Cal
Fat: 31 g
Carbs: 49 g
Protein: 9 g
Fiber: 7 g

BBQ Chickpea and Cauliflower Flatbreads

Preparation Time: 5 minutes
Cooking Time: 15 minutes
Servings: 4
Ingredients:
2 avocados, peeled, pitted, sliced
1 cup BBQ chickpeas
12 ounces chopped cauliflower florets
1 teaspoon salt
2 tablespoons roasted pumpkin seeds, salted
1 tablespoon olive oil
2 tablespoons lemon juice
4 flatbreads, toasted
Hot sauce as needed for serving
Directions:
Place a large baking sheer]t, place cauliflower in it, add oil, season with ¼ teaspoon salt, toss until well coated, and then bake for 25 minutes at 425 degrees F until don't.
Meanwhile, place the avocado in a bowl, add remaining salt and lemon juice, mash well with a fork and then spread on one side of flatbreads.
Distribute roasted cauliflower between flatbreads, top with chickpeas and pumpkin seeds, drizzle with hot sauce and then serve.
Nutrition:
Calories: 500 Cal
Fat: 25 g
Carbs: 65 g
Protein: 11 g
Fiber: 13 g

Summer Minestrone

Preparation Time: 5 minutes
Cooking Time: 15 minutes
Servings: 4
Ingredients:
1 medium yellow squash, cut into 1/2-inch pieces
1/2 cup frozen peas
1 small carrot, peeled, sliced
1 small zucchini, cut into 1/2-inch pieces
8 ounces red potatoes, peeled, cut into 1/2-inch pieces
1 large onion, peeled, chopped
1 tablespoon olive oil
1 teaspoon minced garlic
1/3 teaspoon ground black pepper
2/3 teaspoon salt
1 cup chopped basil
4 cups vegetable broth
1/4 cup grated vegan parmesan cheese
Directions:
Take a large saucepan, place it over medium heat, add oil and when hot, add onion, stir in black pepper and salt and cook for 8 minutes.
Then stir in garlic, cook for 1 minute, stir in potatoes, pour in broth and simmer for 5 minutes.
Add carrot, squash, and zucchini, continue simmer for 3 minutes, and then add peas, simmer for another 3 minutes.
Stir in basil and cheese and then serve with bread.
Nutrition:
Calories: 185 Cal
Fat: 6 g
Carbs: 29 g
Protein: 7 g
Fiber: 5 g

Potatoes with Nacho Sauce

Preparation Time: 10 minutes
Cooking Time: 30 minutes
Servings: 4
Ingredients:
2 pounds mixed baby potatoes, halved
1/2 jalapeno chili, deseeded, chopped
1 cup cashews, soaked, drained
1/2 teaspoon garlic powder
1/2 teaspoon red chili powder
1 teaspoon of sea salt
1/2 teaspoon sweet paprika
1/2 teaspoon ground cumin
1/4 cup nutritional yeast
3 tablespoons lemon juice
3 tablespoons olive oil
1 cup of water
Tortilla chips for serving
Directions:
Place potatoes in a baking sheet, drizzle with oil, season with ½ teaspoon salt and ¼ teaspoon black pepper, and roast for 30 minutes at 450 degrees F until crispy and golden.
Meanwhile, place the remaining ingredients in a blender and pulse for 2 minutes until smooth.
Tip the sauce in a saucepan and cook for 5 minutes at the medium-low level until warm and then serve with roasted potatoes and tortilla chips.
Nutrition:
Calories: 380 Cal
Fat: 18 g
Carbs: 47 g
Protein: 10 g
Fiber: 6 g

Veggie Kabobs

Preparation Time: 10 minutes
Cooking Time: 10 minutes
Servings: 10
Ingredients:
8 ounces button mushrooms, halved
2 pounds summer squash, peeled, 1-inch cubed
12 ounces small broccoli florets
2 cups grape tomatoes
1 teaspoon salt
1/2 teaspoon smoked paprika
1 teaspoon ground cumin
6 tablespoons olive oil
1/2 teaspoon ground coriander
1 lime, juiced
Directions:
Toss broccoli florets with 1 tablespoon oil, toss tomatoes and squash pieces with 2 tablespoons oil, then toss mushrooms with 1 tablespoon oil and thread these vegetables onto skewers.
Grill mushrooms and broccoli for 7 to 10 minutes, squash and tomatoes and 8 minutes, and when done, transfer the skewers to a plate and drizzle with lime juice and remaining oil.
Prepared the spice mix and for this, stir together salt, paprika, cumin, and coriander, sprinkle half of the mixture over grilled veggies, cover them with foil for 5 minutes, and then sprinkle with the remaining spice mix.
Serve straight away.
Nutrition:
Calories: 110 Cal
Fat: 9 g
Carbs: 8 g
Protein: 3 g
Fiber: 3 g

Summer Pesto Pasta

Preparation Time: 10 minutes
Cooking Time: 10 minutes
Servings: 4
Ingredients:
1 pound whole-grain spaghetti, cooked
2 cups grape tomatoes, halved
2 ears corn, shucked
1 medium yellow squash, ½ inch sliced
1 small bell pepper, deseeded, cut into sixths
1 medium zucchini, ½ inch sliced
1/4 cup chopped parsley
4 green onions
1 teaspoon salt
1 teaspoon ground black pepper
1 lemon, juiced, zested
2 tablespoons olive oil
1/2 cup vegan pesto
Directions:
Place corn, onions, bell pepper, zucchini and squash in a bowl, season with ½ teaspoon each of salt and black pepper, and toss until coated.
Grill the corn for 10 minutes, and grill remaining vegetables for 6 minutes until lightly charred and when done, chop vegetables and place them in a bowl.
Place pesto in another bowl, add lemon juice and zest, season with remaining salt and black pepper, and whisk until combined.
Pour pesto over vegetables, toss until mixed, then cut kernels from grilled cobs, add them to the vegetables, then add pasta, parsley, and tomatoes and toss until combined.
Serve straight away.
Nutrition:
Calories: 370 Cal
Fat: 12 g
Carbs: 54 g
Protein: 12 g
Fiber: 5 g

Linguine with Wild Mushrooms

Preparation Time: 5 minutes
Cooking Time: 3 minutes
Servings: 4
Ingredients:
12 ounces mixed mushrooms, sliced
2 green onions, sliced
1 ½ teaspoon minced garlic
1 pound whole-grain linguine pasta, cooked
1/4 cup nutritional yeast
½ teaspoon salt
¾ teaspoon ground black pepper
6 tablespoons olive oil
¾ cup vegetable stock, hot
Directions:
Take a skillet pan, place it over medium-high heat, add garlic and mushroom and cook for 5 minutes until tender.
Transfer the vegetables to a pot, add pasta and remaining ingredients, except for green onions, toss until combined and cook for 3 minutes until hot.
Garnish with green onions and serve.
Nutrition:
Calories: 430 Cal
Fat: 15 g
Carbs: 62 g
Protein: 15 g
Fiber: 5 g

Edamame and Noodle Salad

Preparation Time: 5 minutes
Cooking Time: 5 minutes
Servings: 4
Ingredients:
24 ounces shirataki noodles
1 medium apple, sliced
2 cups grape tomatoes, halved
3 cups frozen edamame, shelled
3 cups shredded carrots
2 cups frozen corn
1/2 teaspoon salt
1/2 cup rice vinegar
1 tablespoon Sriracha hot sauce and more for serving
1/2 cup peanut butter
2 tablespoons water
1/2 cup chopped cilantro
Directions:
Take a large pot, place it over high heat, pour in water, bring it to boil, then add noodles, corn and edamame, boil for 2 minutes and drain when done.
Place remaining ingredients in a large bowl, whisk until combined, then add boiled vegetables and toss until well coated.
Drizzle with more Sriracha sauce and toss until combined.
Nutrition:
Calories: 455 Cal
Fat: 22 g
Carbs: 50 g
Protein: 22 g
Fiber: 13 g

Pilaf with Garbanzos and Dried Apricots

Preparation Time: 10 minutes
Cooking Time: 15 minutes
Servings: 4
Ingredients:
1 cup bulgur
6 ounces cooked chickpeas
1/2 cup Dried apricot
1 small white onion, peeled, diced
½ teaspoon minced garlic
2 teaspoons curry powder
1/2 teaspoon salt
1 tablespoon olive oil
1/4 cup fresh parsley leaves
2 cups vegetable broth
3/4 cup water
Directions:
Take a saucepan, place it over high heat, pour in water and 1 ½ cup broth, and bring it to a boil.
Then stir in bulgur, switch heat to medium-low level and simmer for 15 minutes until most of the liquid has absorbed.
Meanwhile, take a skillet pan, place it over medium heat, add oil and when hot, add onion, cook for 10 minutes, then stir in garlic and curry powder and cook for another minute.
Then add apricots, beans, and salt, pour in remaining broth and bring the mixture to boiling.
Remove pan from heat, fluff the bulgur with a fork, add to the onion-apricot mixture and stir until mixed.
Garnish with parsley and serve.
Nutrition:
Calories: 222 Cal
Fat: 4.5 g
Carbs: 35 g
Protein: 9.5 g
Fiber: 7 g

Avocado and Lime Bean Bowl

Preparation Time: 10 minutes
Cooking Time: 0 minute
Servings: 1
Ingredients:
1/2 cup mint berries
1/4 of medium avocado, pitted, sliced
1/2 cup breakfast beans
12 ounces roasted vegetable mix
1/8 teaspoon salt
1/8 teaspoon cumin
1 teaspoon sunflower seeds
1 teaspoon lime juice
Lime wedges for serving
Directions:
Place avocado in a bowl, mash with a fork and then stir in lime juice, salt, and cumin until combined.
Place roasted vegetable mix in a dish, top with mashed avocado mixture, beans, and sunflower seeds.
Serve with lime wedges and berries.
Nutrition:
Calories: 292 Cal
Fat: 10.4 g
Carbs: 45.6 g
Protein: 9.7 g
Fiber: 12.1 g

Kung Pao Brussels Sprouts

Preparation Time: 10 minutes
Cooking Time: 25 minutes
Servings: 1
Ingredients:
2 pounds Brussels sprouts, halved
1 teaspoon minced garlic
¾ teaspoon ground black pepper
1 tablespoon cornstarch
1 ½ teaspoon salt
1 tablespoon brown sugar
1/8 teaspoon red pepper flakes
1 tablespoon sesame oil
2 tablespoons olive oil
2 teaspoons apple cider vinegar
1/2 cup soy sauce
1 tablespoon hoisin sauce
2 teaspoons garlic chili sauce
1/2 cup water
Sesame seeds as needed for garnish
Green onions as needed for garnish
Chopped roasted peanuts as needed for garnish
Directions:
Place sprouts on a baking sheet, drizzle with oil, season with salt and black pepper, and then bake for 20 minutes at 425 degrees F until crispy and tender.
Meanwhile, take a skillet pan, place it over medium heat, add oil and when hot, add garlic and cook for 1 minute until fragrant.
Then stir in cornstarch and remaining ingredients, except for garnishing ingredients and simmer for 3 minutes, set aside until required.
When Brussel sprouts have roasted, add them to the sauce, toss until mixed and broil for 5 minutes until glazed.
When done, garnish with nuts, sesame seeds, and green onions and then serve.
Nutrition:
Calories: 272 Cal
Fat: 17 g
Carbs: 26 g
Protein: 10 g
Fiber: 7 g

Balsamic-Glazed Roasted Cauliflower

Preparation Time: 10 minutes
Cooking Time: 1 hour and 5 minutes
Servings: 4
Ingredients:
1 large head cauliflower, cut into florets
1/2 pound green beans, trimmed
1 medium red onion, peeled, cut into wedges
2 cups cherry tomatoes
½ teaspoon salt
1/4 cup brown sugar
3 tablespoons olive oil
1 cup balsamic vinegar
2 tablespoons chopped parsley, for garnish
Directions:
Place cauliflower florets in a baking dish, add tomatoes, green beans and onion wedges around it, season with salt, and drizzle with oil.
Pour vinegar in a saucepan, stir in sugar, bring the mixture to a boil and simmer for 15 minutes until reduced by half.
Brush the sauce generously over cauliflower florets and then roast for 1 hour at 400 degrees F until cooked, brushing sauce frequently.
When done, garnish vegetables with parsley and then serve.
Nutrition:
Calories: 86 Cal
Fat: 5.7 g
Carbs: 7.7 g
Protein: 3.1 g
Fiber: 3.3 g

Stuffed Sweet Potato

Preparation Time: 10 minutes
Cooking Time: 45 minutes
Servings: 4
Ingredients:
4.5 pounds sweet potatoes
1/3 cup corn kernels
1 cup chopped kale
1/4 cup diced green onion
3/4 cup diced tomato
½ teaspoon minced garlic
1/2 teaspoon sea salt
1/2 teaspoon chipotle flakes
1/2 teaspoon Dijon mustard
1/2 teaspoon smoked paprika
1/2 teaspoon liquid smoke
1/4 teaspoon ground turmeric
1/2 tablespoon lemon juice
3 tablespoons nutritional yeast
1/3 cup cashews, soaked, drained
1 1/2 cup pasta, cooked
1 cup baked pumpkin puree
1/2 cup vegetable broth
Directions:
Wrap each potato in a foil and then bake for 45 minutes at 375 degrees F until tender.
Meanwhile, prepare the cheese sauce and for this, place pumpkin and cashews in a food processor, add garlic, yeast, salt, paprika, chipotle flakes, liquid smoke, turmeric, mustard, and lemon juice, pour in broth and puree until smooth.
Take a pot, place it over medium-low heat, add prepared sauce, then add remaining ingredients, toss until coated, and cook for 5 minutes until kale has wilted.
Season the mixture with salt and black pepper, then switch heat to the low level and cook until sweet potatoes have roasted.
When sweet potatoes are roasted, let them stand for 10 minutes, then unwrap them, split them by slicing down the center and spoon prepared sauce generously in the center.
Serve straight away.
Nutrition:
Calories: 330 Cal
Fat: 3.5 g
Carbs: 58 g
Protein: 13 g
Fiber: 15.2 g

Split Pea Pesto Stuffed Shells

Preparation Time: 15 minutes
Cooking Time: 60 minutes
Servings: 6
Ingredients:
12 ounces jumbo pasta shells, whole-grain, cooked
Marinara sauce as needed for serving
For the Split Pea Pesto:
1 cup green split peas
1/4 cup basil leaves
1 teaspoon minced garlic
1 teaspoon of sea salt
2 tablespoons lemon juice
2 1/4 cups water, divided
Directions:
Take a small saucepan, place it over high heat, add peas, pour in 2 cups water, and bring the beans to boil.
Switch heat to the low level, simmer beans for 30 minutes, and when done, drain the beans then transfer them to a food processor.
Pour in remaining ingredients for the pesto and pulse until blended.
Take a baking dish, spread the marinara sauce in the bottom, then stuffed shell with prepared pesto, arrange them into the prepared baking dish, spread with some marinara sauce over the top and bake for 30 minutes until heated.
Garnish with basil and serve.
Nutrition:
Calories: 82 Cal
Fat: 0 g
Carbs: 15 g
Protein: 6 g
Fiber: 6 g

Tofu Tikka Masala

Preparation Time: 10 minutes
Cooking Time: 4 hours and 10 minutes
Servings: 4
Ingredients:
16 ounces tofu, extra-firm, drained, ½ inch cubed
1 ½ teaspoon minced garlic
2 medium carrots, peeled sliced
1 medium white onion, peeled, diced
1 1/2 cups diced potatoes
1 medium red bell pepper, cored, cut into chunks
¾ cup frozen peas
2 cups cauliflower florets
½ tablespoon grated ginger
¼ teaspoon ground black pepper
½ teaspoon salt
½ teaspoon ground turmeric
1 ½ teaspoons cumin
¼ teaspoon cayenne pepper
1 tablespoon garam masala
1 teaspoon coriander
¼ teaspoon paprika
½ tablespoon maple syrup
15 ounces tomato sauce
15 ounces of coconut milk
2 tablespoons chopped cilantro
Directions:
Take a slow cooker, place all the ingredients in it, except for cilantro and peas, and stir until combined.
Switch on the slow cooker, shut with lid, and cook for 4 hours at a high heat setting.
When done, stir in peas, cook for 10 minutes, uncovering the cooker, and, when done, serve with cooked brown rice.
Nutrition:
Calories: 303 Cal
Fat: 11.5 g
Carbs: 36 g
Protein: 15 g
Fiber: 8.7 g

Conclusion

As an athlete, it may sound like the vegan diet may not provide you the right nutrition. But I am sure after reading these recipes; you can very well debunk that myth.

Over the course of the book, I've given you a bunch of tasty and easy to cook recipes which will make sure that you get your share of protein and carbs. Remember that while being a meat free athlete ain't easy, this is hardly a reason to quit!

One of the greatest benefits of going vegan is the increased level of health you will experience and this manifests well beyond just your physique. Add to this the potent combination of healthy plant based protein and you have a winner! The vegan diet is famous for its health benefits and especially for weight loss. Many people have made a vegan diet to lose weight and have succeeded.

Lose weight, enjoy more energy, and feel good by making a difference in vegetarianism. But before starting a vegan diet, you may be looking for a healthy and healthy diet to lose weight, and there are some things you should understand.

Most people make the mistake of giving the word 'diet' a negative connotation. It is for this reason that most of them are unable to stick to a diet when they want to switch to a different lifestyle. It is important that you do not do that. Tell yourself that you are switching to a healthier lifestyle that has numerous benefits. Remember that it is okay to give yourself one cheat meal. You can consume this meal on those days when you have cravings. You should remember to never make a habit out of it. Once you begin to lead a vegan lifestyle fully, you will no longer have any meat cravings.

To be well prepared, the key is to have an unmistakable objective for the occasion, stick to individual plans and readiness procedures, remain at the time, and limit the effect of interruptions. Staying positive and hopeful, even despite misfortune, and overseeing feelings every day are extra tips that can have a major effect once rivalry shows up. For the groups who are set up for the experience, rivalries give energizing chances to exhibit capacities and are significant learning open doors for youthful athletes.

Now that you have learned the benefits of switching to a vegan lifestyle, and understand that there are ample plant-based or nut-based proteins that can help you provide your body with the necessary protein and other nutrients, it is time for you to get started with the recipes.

www.ingramcontent.com/pod-product-compliance
Lightning Source LLC
Chambersburg PA
CBHW081306250726

48662CB00008B/2423